Recent Results in Cancer Research   167

Managing Editors
P. M. Schlag, Berlin · H.-J. Senn, St. Gallen

Associate Editors
P. Kleihues, Zürich · F. Stiefel, Lausanne
B. Groner, Frankfurt · A. Wallgren, Göteborg

Founding Editor
P. Rentchnik, Geneva

C. Stroszczynski (Ed.)

Minimally Invasive Tumor Therapies

With 43 Figures and 21 Tables

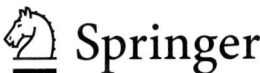

Priv.-Doz. Dr. med. Christian Stroszczynski
Faculty of Medicine Carl Gustav Carus
University Hospital
Departement of Diagnostic Radiology
Fetscherstrasse 74
01377 Dresden
Germany
email: stros@uniklinikum-dresden.de

Library of Congress Control Number: 2006921644
ISSN 0080-0015
ISBN 10 3-540-28136-3   Springer Berlin Heidelberg New York
ISBN 13 978-3-540-28136-8   Springer Berlin Heidelberg New York

This work is subject to copyright. All rights reserved, whether the whole or part of the material is concerned, specifically the rights of translation, reprinting, reuse of illustrations, recitation, broadcasting, reproduction on microfilm or in any other way, and storage in databanks. Duplication of this publication or parts thereof is permitted only under the provisions of the German Copyright Law of September, 9, 1965, in its current version, and permission for use must always be obtained from Springer-Verlag. Violations are liable for prosecution under the German Copyright Law.

Springer is a part of Springer Science + Business Media
springeronline.com

© Springer-Verlag Berlin Heidelberg 2006

The use of general descriptive names, registered names, trademarks, etc. in this publication does not imply, even in the absence of a specific statement, that such names are exempt from the relevant protective laws and regulations and therefore free for general use.
Product liability: The publisher cannot guarantee the accuracy of any information about dosage and application contained in this book. In every individual case the user must check such information by consulting the relevant literature.

Editor: Dr. Ute Heilmann, Heidelberg
Desk editor: Dörthe Mennecke-Bühler, Heidelberg
Cover design: Frido Steinen Broo, eStudio Calamar, Spain
Production & Typesetting: LE-TEX Jelonek, Schmidt & Vöckler GbR, Leipzig
Printed on acid-free paper   11528944   21/3150/YL – 5 4 3 2 1 0

Contents

Part I   Image Guidance of Minimally Invasive Tumor Therapies

1   Use of Imaging Modalities for the Guidance of Minimally Invasive Tumor Therapies (MITT) 3
Christian Stroszczynski, Gunnar Gaffke

2   Development of Navigation Systems for Image-Guided Laparoscopic Tumor Resections in Liver Surgery 13
Thomas Lange, Michael Hünerbein, Sebastian Eulenstein, Sigfried Beller, Peter Michael Schlag

Part II   Methods of Minimally Invasive Tumor Therapies

3   Radiofrequency Ablation: The Percutaneous Approach 39
Philippe Pereira, Andreas Boss, Stephen Clasen, Cecile Gouttefangeas, Diethard Schmidt, Claus D. Claussen

4   The Surgical Approach for Radiofrequency Ablation of Liver Tumors 53
Guido Schumacher, Robert Eisele, Antonino Spinelli, Peter Neuhaus

5   Laser-Induced Thermotherapy 69
Birger Mensel, Christiane Weigel, Norbert Hosten

Part III   Clinical Results of Minimally Invasive Tumor Therapies

6   Liver Metastases 79
Andreas Lubienski, Thorsten Leibecke, Karin Lubienski, Thomas Helmberger

7	**Percutaneous Ablation of Hepatocellular Carcinoma**	91
	Riccardo Lencioni, Clodilde Della Pina, Laura Crocetti, Dania Cioni	
8	**Lung Tumors**	107
	K. Steinke	
9	**Renal Tumors**	123
	Andreas Mahnken, Joseph Tacke	
10	**Thermal Ablation in Bone Tumors**	135
	Bernhard Gebauer, Per-Ulf Tunn	

List of Contributors

Dr. med. Bernhard Gebauer
Dept. of Radiology
Charité – Campus Buch
HELIOS-Klinikum
Lindenberger Weg 80
13125 Berlin
Germany

Professor Dr. med. Norbert Hosten
Klinikum der Ernst-Moritz-Arndt-Universität
Klinik und Poliklinik für Radiologie
Fr.-Loeffler-Str. 23
17487 Greifswald
Germany

Dr. med. Thomas Lange
Klinik für Chirurgie
und Chirurgische Onkologie
Robert-Rössle-Klinik
Lindenberger Weg 80
13122 Berlin
Germany

Professor Dr. Riccardo Lencioni
Division of Diagnostic
and Interventional Radiology
University of Pisa
Via Roma 67
I-56125 Pisa
Italy

Dr. med. A. Lubienski
Institute of Radiology
University Hospital Schleswig-Holstein
Campus Lübeck
Ratzeburger Allee 160
23538 Lübeck
Germany

Dr. med. Andreas H. Mahnken
Department of Diagnostic Radiology
University Hospital, RWTH Aachen University
Pauwelsstraße 30
52074 Aachen
Germany

Professor Philippe L. Pereira
Professor and Research Director of Radiology
Division of Local Therapy
Vice-Chairman of the Department
of Diagnostic Radiology
Hoppe-Seyler-Str. 3
72076 Tübingen
Germany

Dr. med. Guido Schumacher
Dept. of General, Visceral,
and Transplantation Surgery
Charité Campus Virchow-Klinikum
Augustenburger Platz 1
13353 Berlin
Germany

PD Dr. med. Karin Steinke
Universitätsspital Basel
CH-4031 Basel
Switzerland

Priv.-Doz. Dr. med. Christian Stroszczynski
Faculty of Medicine Carl Gustav Carus
University Hospital
Departement of Diagnostic Radiology
Fetscherstrasse 74
01377 Dresden
Germany

Dr. med. Christiane Weigel
Ernst-Moritz-Arndt-Universität
Sauerbruchstr.
17487 Greifswald
Germany

Part I Image Guidance of Minimally Invasive Tumor Therapies

Use of Imaging Modalities for the Guidance of Minimally Invasive Tumor Therapies (MITT)

Christian Stroszczynski, Gunnar Gaffke

1.1 Staging

The decision on whether a regional therapy might induce a benefit for the patient should be based on staging that is as precise as possible. While surgical exploration, palpation, and intraoperative ultrasound have been the gold standard for the detection of distant metastases, the number of patients with small distant metastases in liver, lung, and bone identified by computed tomography, magnetic resonance imaging, and positron emission tomography that cannot be visualized intraoperatively is increasing, reflecting the progress of imaging methods over the last few years (Antoch et al. 2003; Bhattacharjya et al. 2004a). When minimally invasive tumor therapies (MITT) are used, the intervention has to be planned based on imaging alone or combined with a focal exploration such as laparoscopy or video-assisted thoracoscopy. Staging based on imaging alone might induce inappropriate therapy in cases of false-negative or false positive-findings, indicating that highly accurate imaging methods are of crucial importance for the planning of image-guided therapies.

On the other hand, the accuracy of imaging methods is still limited for the differentiation of lymphonodal involvement as well as for diffuse tumor infiltrations, i.e., peritoneal carcinomatosis (Antoch et al. 2004). Usually, minimally invasive tumor therapies are used in patients with localized relapse of cancer, involving precise staging where further tumor activity may be excluded by imaging methods. Positron emission tomography using fluorodeoxyglucose (FDG-PET) without or combined with computed tomography has been established as the most sensitive imaging modality for the detection of additional tumor manifestations for various types of cancer (Barker et al. 2005; Bipat et al. 2005). Because of the relatively high primary costs and a variable regional availability, only a few patients had PET or PET-CT when they were evaluated for regional tumor therapies. Whole-body MRI has been established during the last 5 years with promising preliminary results for the staging of cancer patients (Blomqvist and Torkzad 2004). Several technical developments have led to the acquisition time for large fields of view being reduced significantly. Whole-body MR imaging protocols can be performed in less than 40 min, making this method attractive for use in daily clinical practice. Whole-body MRI can be combined with organ-specific contrast media such as superparamagnetic iron oxides and hepatobiliary contrast agents with the intention to establish entity-specific protocols in the near future (Semelka and Thermberger 2001). However, there is still a need for systematic and comparative studies for whole-body MRI in oncology. More than 90% of minimally invasive tumor therapies are performed on liver tumors (Gazelle et al. 2000; Bown 1983). Several liver-specific MR contrast media are now established in clinical practice. Reticuloendothelial system-specific agents improve lesion detection by decreasing the signal intensity of background liver on T2-weighted MR images, which increases the conspicuity of focal hepatic lesions with negligible reticuloendothelial cells (e.g., metastases). Hepatocyte-selective agents increase the signal intensity of background liver on T1-weighted images, which increases the conspicuity of focal lesions that do not contain hepatocytes (e.g., metastases). Several studies have demonstrated a better lesion-based sensitivity of MRI for liver metastases using liver-specific contrast media when compared with CT (Fig. 1.1). However, computed tomography is still the method of choice for the staging of most of the patients in clinical routine because of its versatility (Semelka and Thermberger 2001; Bhattacharjya et al. 2004b). Oncologic CT imaging protocols should include the examination of the liver in several phases, especially when local therapy of liver tumors should be evaluated.

1.2 Image Guidance

For image-guidance of minimal invasive tumor therapies, ultrasound, computed tomography, and magnetic resonance imaging can be used. Most surgeons and some radiologists, particularly in the United States and Italy, prefer ultrasound (US), while CT is the method of choice for radiologists in several European countries (Gazelle et al. 2000; Tranberg et al. 1994; Vogl et al. 1995; Gaffke et al. 2005).

Ultrasound can be used for image-guided therapies of the liver but cannot be used for interventions of the lung or the bone because of its technical limitations. For image-guided therapies of the liver, ultrasound is widely used because of its good availability, low cost, multiplanarity, and the easiness of handling. Percutaneous use of US for image-guided therapy of the liver is sometimes hampered by reduced image quality due to obesity or inhomogeneous echogenicity of the organ. In addition, the use of US is less favorable for complex image-guided interventions,

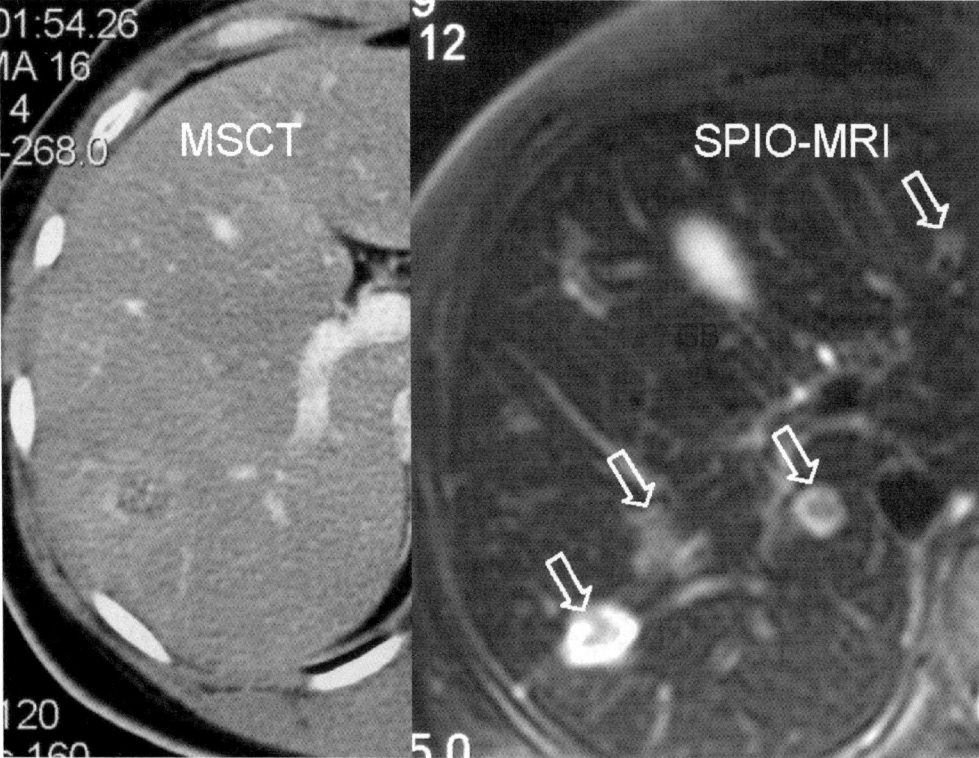

Fig. 1.1 CT and SPIO-MRI of a patient with liver metastases evaluated for minimally invasive tumor therapies. While CT shows poor visualization of liver metastases, MRI using SPIO as liver-specific contrast media demonstrates clearly four hyperintense liver lesions (GB: gallbladder)

i.e., multiapplicator techniques and step-by-step ablations of larger tumors, because of relevant artifacts induced by air that may brought in during intervention or nitrogen bubbles that occur during thermoablative procedures (Fig. 1.2).

Many radiologists who have access to all imaging modalities prefer CT for image-guided therapy (Vogl et al. 1995; Mahnken et al. 2005; Gaffke et al. 2006). In contrast to ultrasound, both hands can be used for interventional procedures and CT is suitable for intervention in all regions of the body. In addition, complications that may be provoked during intervention such as intra-abdominal bleeding or pneumothoraces can be visualized before clinical signs occur. CT fluoroscopy enabling quasi real-time imaging has been established since the end of the 1990s in many hospitals as being of significant impact for difficult or complex interventions (Fig. 1.3). While diagnostic CT is usually performed with contrast media using arterial, portovenous and venous phases for the detection and differentiation of liver tumors, CT-guided interventions are performed on plain images. Lesion-based sensitivity of plain CT for liver tumors is poor. In daily clinical practice, the exact position of the applicators must be controlled by contrast-enhanced images during interventions in most cases. In most cases, a sufficient contrast between target lesion and liver tissue can be obtained in a few seconds and repetitive contrast media application is limited by nephrotoxicity. A permanent increase of liver-to-lesion contrast in hepatocellular carcinoma and other hypervascularized tumors can be obtained by intra-arterial application of iodized oil (iodized oil CT, IOCT). However, IOCT has not been established in clinical practice and has its limitation in patients with hypovascular tumors, i.e., liver metastases of most of gastrointestinal tumors and breast tumors (Bhattacharjya et al. 2004a). Because of this limitation, some groups have established a hybrid procedure using CT for the positioning of the applicators in the environment of the tumor and the closed MRI-scanner for multiplanar control of the position, eventually combined

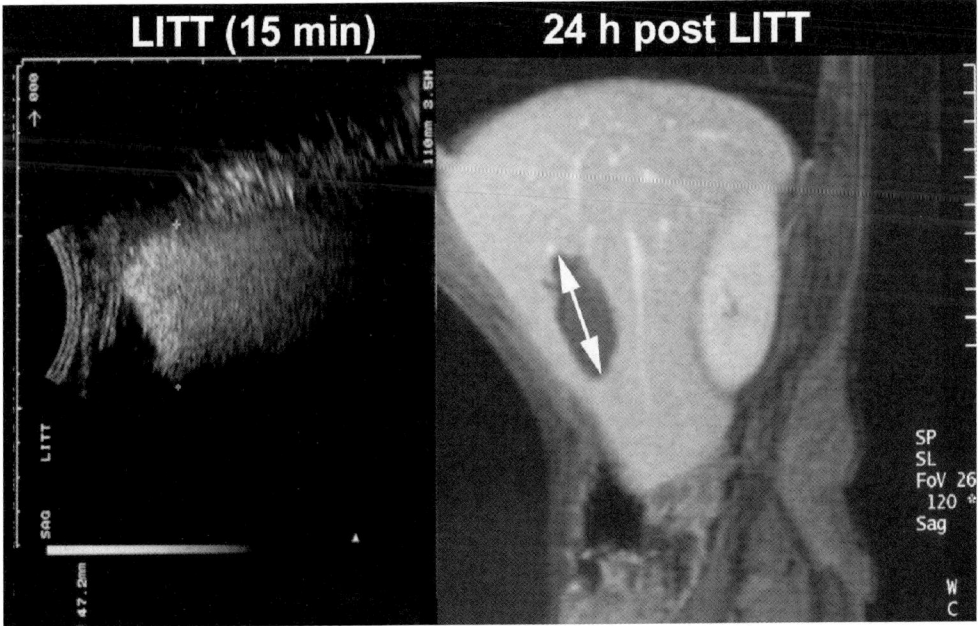

Fig. 1.2 Ultrasound during laser therapy of a liver metastasis and corresponding MRI, both on sagittal orientation. The hyperechogenic area visualized on US is provoked by nitrogen bubbles that occur during tissue heating. US tends to overestimate ablation zone, as demonstrated on postinterventional MRI

with a repositioning in the magnet (Vogl et al. 1995; Gaffke et al. 2006).

Image-guided therapy in closed high-field MRI units is possible (Puls et al. 2003), but time-consuming and often narrowed by the limited space in the MR scanner with a small gantry (Fig. 1.4). Open MRI scanners or MRI with larger gantries enable more comfortable positioning of the applicators (Aschoff et al. 2000). When compared with CT, open MRI seems to be a promising tool for MITT in the nearer future because of the availability of multiplanar near real-time images (MR fluoroscopy) and an optimal, permanent contrast between lesions and normal tissue.

1.3 Thermometry

Until recently, thermoablative therapies were often performed without visual control of the induced temperature. Many factors influence the size of induced necrosis by thermal ablation techniques (i.e., tissue perfusion, heat conduction) and prevent precise prediction of the size of induced necrosis (Dickinson et al. 1986; Wlodarcyk et al. 1998). Some authors used ultrasound to visualize thermal effects during tissue heating. For cryotherapy, excellent visualization of the induced ice ball is possible by ultrasound. In contrast, thermomapping of heated tissue is not possible with ultrasound (Morrison et al. 2000). There is a certain correlation between the appearance of hyperechogenic areas that are provoked by nitrogen bubbles in tissue heated to over 60 °C, but these areas do not precisely correlate with the areas where a complete ablation is obtained and may simulate a successful ablation despite incomplete heating (Stroszczynski et al. 2002).

Therefore, several authors use thermosensitive MR sequences for immediate MR temperature monitoring. MR thermometry can be performed precisely using specialized MR sequences in all

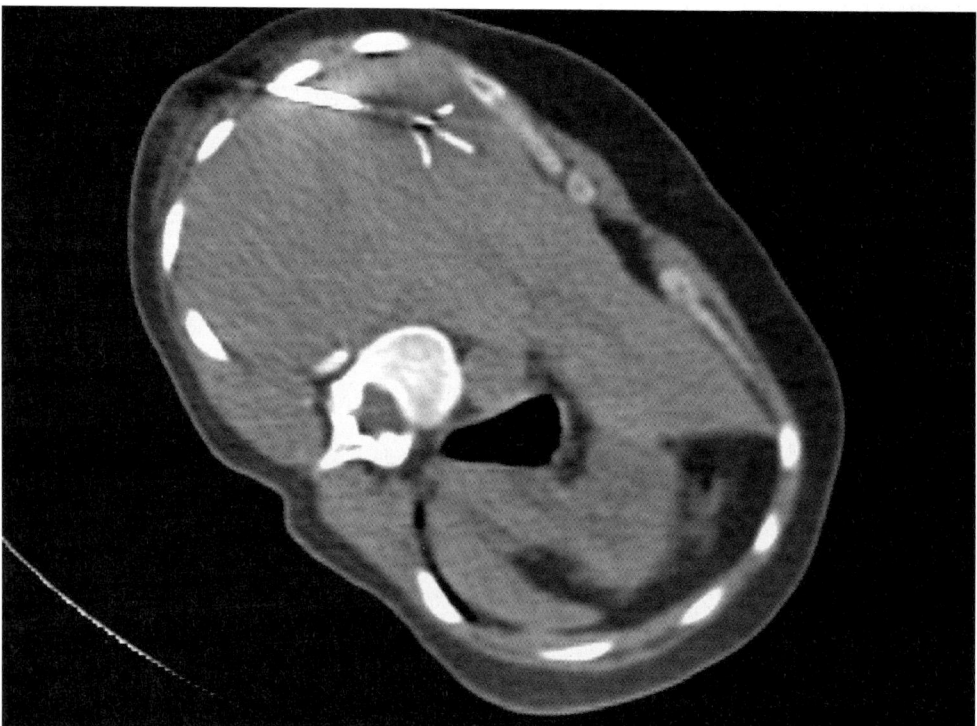

Fig. 1.3 CT fluoroscopy during radiofrequency ablation of a liver tumor

kinds of tissue, i.e., liver, breast, pancreas, and brain (Fig. 1.5) (Matsumoto et al. 1994; Kahn et al. 1998; Olsrud et al. 1998; Stroszczynski et al. 2001). When compared with brain tissue or liver tissue, the temperature monitoring of thermal interventions of the lung is more pretentious because of the susceptibility of surrounding gut and multiple sources of different artifacts. For thermometry, MR-compatible devices are necessary. While laser therapy and cryoablation can be performed during the heating or cooling process, radiofrequency ablation cannot be visualized online because of relevant artifacts induced by the radiofrequency generator. However, sufficient differentiation between devitalized tissue and residual tumor is possible using hyperacute MRI immediately after heating by radiofrequency. In cases of incomplete ablation, the immediate repositioning of the RF device is possible and additional applications may follow (Merkle et al. 1999; Gaffke et al. 2005).

Although proton resonance frequency or diffusion weighted images are more accurate for thermometry in vitro, the T1 method using a FLASH sequence is preferred by several groups because of a high level of robustness (Wlodarcyk et al. 1998). Several investigators used temperature-sensitive sequences to reduce the risk of damage of critical structures for thermoablation of liver neoplasms or brain tumors (Gewiese et al. 1994; Kahn et al. 1998).

1.4 Therapy Control

Currently, thermoablative techniques such as laser therapy or radiofrequency ablation are being introduced into clinical practice for the treatment of liver tumors. Based on the analysis of data acquired from liver surgery, a significant impact on survival may be expected in patients with complete tumor ablation only (Scheele and Altendorf-Hofmann 1999). In contrast to surgery, where histopathology enables quality control of

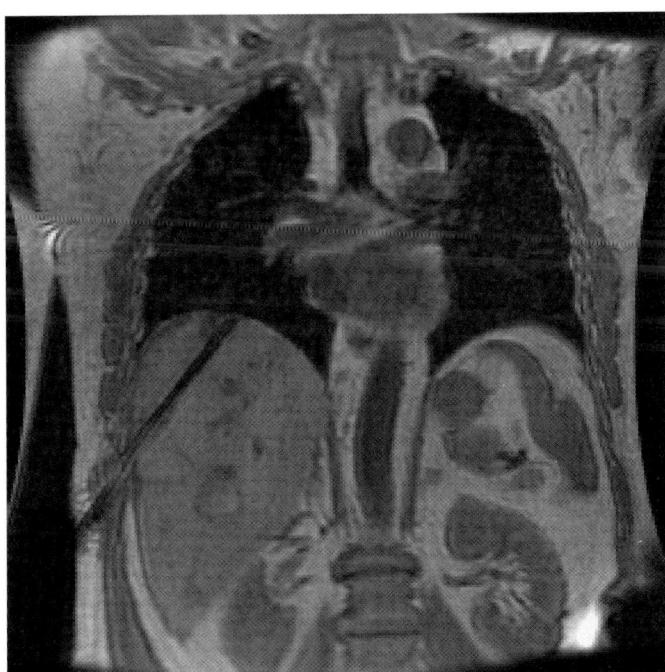

Fig. 1.4 MR-guided radiofrequency ablation of a liver metastasis using a closed high-field scanner. Coronal orientation provides an optimal overview of critical structures such as the costodiaphragmatic angle

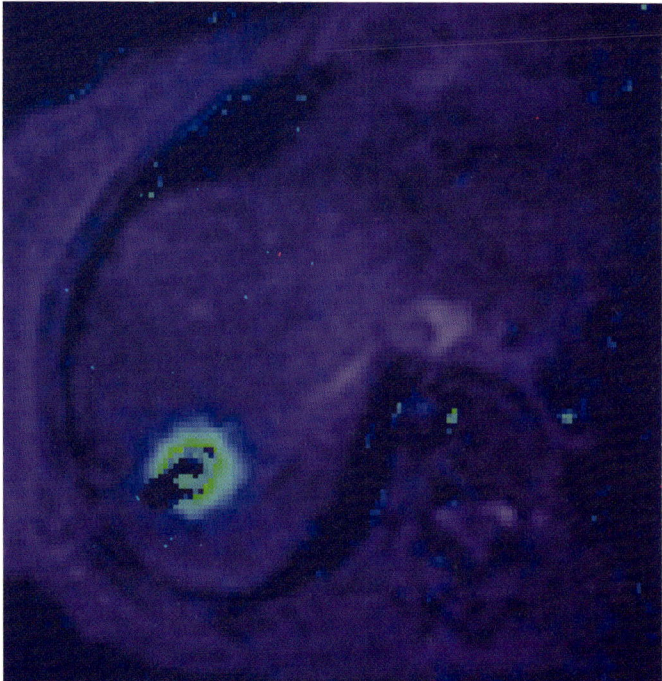

Fig. 1.5 Color-coded temperature mapping during laser therapy of a liver lesion

resection of liver tumors, precise postinterventional imaging is necessary after thermoablative techniques to visualize residual tumor.

To differentiate therapy-induced necrosis from residual tumor, ultrasound, computed tomography, magnetic resonance imaging, and positron emission tomography can be used (Germer et al. 1998; Veit et al. 2006). Therapy-induced necrosis is characterized by low concentrations of water-bounded protons, the absence of blood perfusion, and hypometabolism. In residual tumor tissue, neoangiogenic vessels with capillary leakage induce peripheral edema and cause enhancement of conventional contrast media (Choi et al. 2000). In addition, the tumors show highly proliferative activity and glucose uptake that can be measured by different PET tracers (Veit et al. 2006).

Some groups use MRI for the differentiation between residual tumor and therapy-induced necrosis because of the excellent contrast and spatial resolution in soft tissue (Morrison et al. 1998). Coagulation of tumor or liver tissue leads to tissue drying and results in hypointense lesions on T2-weighted images, while residual tumor is usually hyperintense caused by tumor edema (Semelka et al. 2000; Stroszczynski et al. 2001). When conventional extracellular contrast media such as Gd-DTPA are used, T1-W images may differentiate between vascularized residual tumor and nonperfused necrosis (Vogl et al. 1995). Liver-specific contrast media such as superparamagnetic iron oxides that enhance in the reticular endothelial system or Gd-EOB or Gd-BOPTA that enhance in healthy hepatocytes may increase contrast between normal liver tissue and thermal-induced necrosis or residual tumor. However, the use of so-called liver specific contrast media does not increase the contrast between residual tumor and thermoablative scar, because liver-specific contrast media only accumulates in healthy liver tissue.

Using healthy animal models, correlations of MRI findings after thermoablation of normal liver tissue on T2-W, plain, and early (0.2- to 10-min) enhanced T1-W images with histopathology were investigated by Germer and Coworkers. Characteristics for complete devitalized liver tissue are hypointensity on T2-W images and the lack of enhancement on early-enhanced (0.2- to

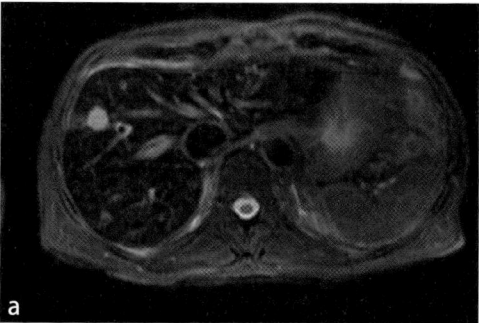 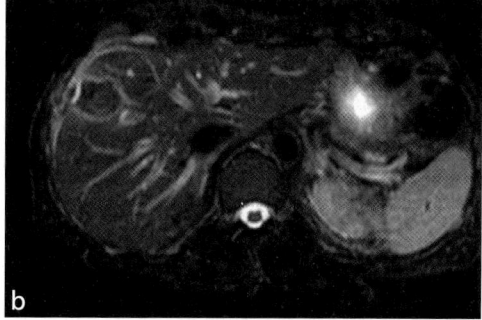

Fig. 1.6 a MRI of a patient with solitary liver metastasis of an adenocarcinoma. T2-W images demonstrated a highly hyperintense tumor because of a high concentration of water-bounded protons in the tumor. b Five days after radiofrequency ablation, the signal intensity of the tumor and the surrounding tissue is reduced because of coagulation and complete necrosis of the treated area. A small hyperintense rim caused by inflammation around the necrotic area is visible

10-min) T1-W images (Fig. 1.6). In contrast to animal studies, inconclusive or discordant findings on postinterventional MRI are common in clinical practice because of several additional parameters influencing signal intensity of treated areas (i.e., residual tumor, bleeding, injection of fibrin gluen and local anesthesia).

Germer et al. systematically correlated MR pattern after i.v. administration of conventional doses of Gd-DTPA (0.1 mmol/kg) of early-enhanced images after LITT of normal livers in 55 rabbits with histomorphologic findings. They observed three zones on MRI and histopathology: the coagulation zone (zone with completely damaged liver tissue), the small transition zone located between the central zone and the undamaged liver tissue, and the reference zone surrounding the lesion with undamaged liver tissue. Early-enhanced MRI correlated well with that obtained macroscopically ($r = 0.96$). Both the central zone and transition zone did not enhance Gd-DTPA 24 h after LITT on early-enhanced images. However, the transition zone reflecting a zone where residual tumor cells may be found measured approximately 2 mm and may be neglected in clinical practice. In contrast to findings of Aschoff and co-workers, lesions of patients with complete ablation were significantly larger on T2-W images on this study, indicating the limited value of this sequence for early postinterventional control.

Late-enhanced MRI 10 min to 6 h after administration of extracellular contrast media (Gd-DTPA) is considered as to be specific for necrotic tissue, i.e., for myocardial infarction (Ni et al. 2001) and could be used for imaging of necrotic areas. Mechanisms of delayed enhancement in devitalized tissue have remained unclear until now. Similar to the hypothesis concerning the uptake of metalloporphyrins, active protein binding of the macrocyclic extracellular Gd complexes in the transition zone with or without consecutive alteration of T1-relaxivity could be a possible cause for delayed enhancement. These findings might be of importance for early postinterventional therapy planning.

Recently, positron emission tomography (PET) without or combined with computed tomography (PET/CT) using [F-18] fluorodeoxyglucose (FDG) has been investigated for the evaluation of liver metastases after radiofrequency ablation and other interstitial tumor therapies. FDG PET and PET/CT can provide added diagnostic information compared with conventional imaging in patients after radiofrequency ablation of liver metastases and can be useful in guiding repeat ablation procedures (Veit et al. 2006). PET/CT therefore possibly proved superior to CT alone when assessing the liver for residual tumor after RFA. However, false-negative results may occur using PET/CT hidden by normal FDG-uptake in surrounding normal liver tissue. The most sensitive approach detecting residual disease in liver treated by minimally invasive tumor therapies seems to be a combined use of MRI and FDG-PET. While PET-MRI scanners have not been available until now, retrospective fusion of MRI and PET data can be easily done based on commercially available software tools. The most important supplementary finding supplied by image fusion is a more precise correlation with focal tracer hot spots in PET (Fig. 1.7).

References

1. Antoch G, Vogt FM, Freudenberg LS, Nazaradeh F, Goehde SC, Barkhausen J, Dahmen G, Bockisch A, Debatin JF, Ruehm SG (2003) Whole-body dual-modality PET/CT and whole-body MRI for tumor staging in oncology. JAMA 290:3199–3206

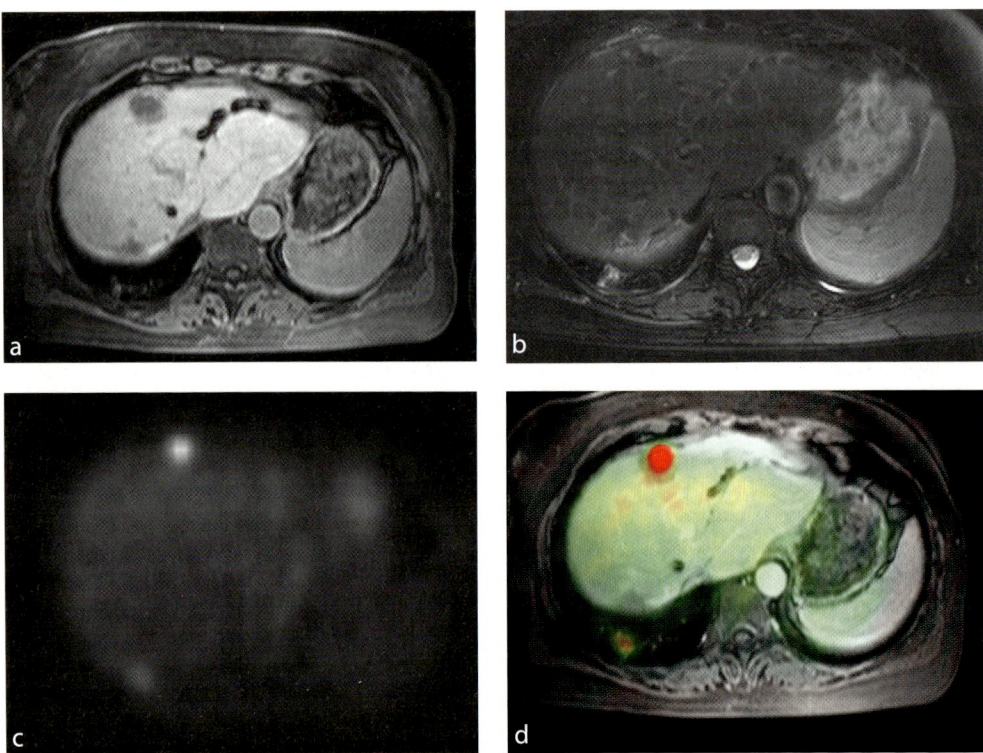

Fig. 7 a Contrast-enhanced MRI of a patient with colorectal cancer and hemihepatectomy. Two new liver metastases were treated by radiofrequency ablation (RFA) 6 months ago. MRI was performed because of rising CEA level during follow-up. Contrast enhanced T1-W images demonstrate two hypointense scars after RFA. **b** On T2-W images, a hyperintense area close to the ventral scar is visualized, suggesting local recurrence. In addition, a hyperintense focal lung lesion is visible. **c** FDG-PET on axial orientation shows two hypermetabolic areas, both suggesting tumor activity. It remains unclear if the second focus is located in the lung or in the liver (Courtesy of Dr. Dresel, Chairman of the Dept. of Nuclear Medicine Robert-Rössle Klinik Charité Campus Buch). **d** Fusion of FDG-PET and MRI underlines local recurrence in the ventral liver lesion and the appearance of the new lung metastases. In contrast, no activity is visualized in the second liver lesion

2. Antoch G, Saoudi N, Kuehl H, Dahmen G, Mueller SP, Beyer T, Bockisch A, Debatin JF, Freudenberg LS (2004) Accuracy of whole-body dual-modality fluorine-18-2-fluoro-2-deoxy-D-glucose positron emission tomography and computed tomography (FDG-PET/CT) for tumor staging in solid tumors: comparison with CT and PET. J Clin Oncol 22:4357–4368
3. Aschoff AJ, Rafie N, Jesberger JA et al. (2000) Thermal lesion conspicuity following interstitial radiofrequency thermal tumor ablation in humans: a comparison of STIR, turbo spin-echo T2-weighted, and contrast-enhanced T1-weighted MR images at 0.2 T. J Magn Reson Imaging 12:584–589
4. Barker DW, Zagoria RJ, Morton KA, Kavanagh PV, Shen P (2005) Evaluation of liver metastases after radiofrequency ablation: utility of 18F-FDG PET and PET/CT. Am J Roentgenol 184:1096–1102
5. Bhattacharjya S, Bhattacharjya T, Baber S, Tibballs JM, Watkinson AF, Davidson BR (2004a) Prospective study of contrast-enhanced computed tomography, computed tomography during arterioportography, and magnetic resonance imaging for staging colorectal liver metastases for liver resection. Br J Surg 91:1361–1369
6. Bhattacharjya S, Bhattacharjya T, Quaglia A, Dhillon AP, Burroughs AK, Patch DW, Tibballs JM, Watkinson AF, Rolles K, Davidson BR (2004b) Liver transplantation in cirrhotic patients with small hepatocellular carcinoma: an analysis of pre-operative imaging, explant histology and prognostic histologic indicators. Dig Surg 21:152–159
7. Bipat S, van Leeuwen MS, Comans EF, Pijl ME, Bossuyt PM, Zwinderman AH, Stoker J (2005) Colorectal liver metastases: CT, MR imaging, and PET for diagnosis-meta-analysis. Radiology 237:123–131
8. Blomqvist L, Torkzad MR (2004) Whole-body imaging with MRI or PET/CT: the future for single-modality imaging in oncology? JAMA 290:3248–3249
9. Bown SG (1983) Phototherapy of tumors. World J Surg 7:700–709
10. Choi SI, Jiang CZ, Lim KH et al. (2000) Application of breath-hold T2-weighted, first-pass perfusion and gadolinium-enhanced T1-weighted MR imaging for assessment of myocardial viability in a pig model. J Magn Reson Imaging 11:476–480
11. Dickinson RJ, Hall AS, Hind AJ, Young IR (1986) Measurement of changes in tissue temperature using MR imaging. J Comp Assist Tomogr 10:468–472
12. Gaffke G, Gebauer B, Gnauck M, Knollmann F, Helmberger T, Ricke J, Oettle H, Felix R, Stroszczynski C (2005) Potential advantages of the MRI for the radiofrequency ablation of liver tumors. Fortschr Rontgenstr 177:77–84
13. Gaffke G, Gebauer B, Knollmann FD, Helmberger T, Ricke J, Oettle H, Felix R, Stroszczynski C (2006) Use of semiflexible applicators for radiofrequency ablation of liver tumors. Cardiovasc Intervent Radiol 29:270–275
14. Gazelle GS, Goldberg SN, Solbiati L, Livraghi T (2000) Tumor ablation with radio-frequency energy. Radiology 217:633–646
15. Germer CT, Isbert CM, Albrecht D et al. (1998) Laser-induced thermotherapy for the treatment of liver metastasis: correlation of gadolinium-DTPA-enhanced MRI with histomorphologic findings to determine criteria for follow-up monitoring. Surg Endosc 12:1317–1325
16. Gewiese B, Beuthan J, Fobbe F, Stiller D, Mueller G, Boese-Landgraf J, Wolf KJ, Deimling M (1994) Magnetic resonance imaging-controlled laser-induced interstitial thermotherapy. Invest Radiol 29:345–351
17. Kahn T, Harth T, Kiwit JC, Schwarzmaier HJ, Wald C, Modder U (1998) In vivo MRI thermometry using a phase-sensitive sequence: preliminary experience during MRI-guided laser-induced interstitial thermotherapy of brain tumors. J Magn Reson Imaging 8:160–164
18. Mahnken AH, Rohde D, Brkovic D, Gunther RW, Tacke JA (2005). Percutaneous radiofrequency ablation of renal cell carcinoma: preliminary results. Acta Radiol 46:208–214
19. Matsumoto R, Mulkern RV, Hushek SG, Jolesz FA (1994) Tissue temperature monitoring for thermal interventional therapy: comparison of T1-weighted MR sequences. J Magn Reson Imaging 4:65–70
20. Merkle EM, Haaga JR, Duerk JL, Jacobs GH, Brambs HJ, Lewin JS (1999) MR imaging-guided radio-frequency thermal ablation in the pancreas in a porcine model with a modified clinical C-arm system. Radiology 213:461–467

21. Morrison PR, Jolesz FA, Charous D et al. (1998) MRI of laser-induced interstitial thermal injury in an in vivo animal liver model with histologic correlation. J Magn Reson Imaging 18:57–63
22. Ni Y, Pislaru C, Bosmans H et al. (2001) Intracoronary delivery of Gd-DTPA and Gadophrin-2 for determination of myocardial viability with MR imaging. Eur Radiol 11:876–883
23. Olsrud J, Wirestam R, Brockstedt S, Nilsson AM, Tranberg KG, Stahlberg F, Persson BR (1998) MRI thermometry in phantoms by use of the proton resonance frequency shift method: application to interstitial laser thermotherapy. Phys Med Biol 43:2597–2613
24. Puls R, Stroszczynski C, Gaffke G, Hosten N, Felix R, Speck U (2003) Laser-induced thermotherapy (LITT) of liver metastases: MR-guided percutaneous insertion of an MRI-compatible irrigated microcatheter system using a closed high-field unit. J Magn Reson Imaging 17:663–670
25. Scheele J, Altendorf-Hofmann A (1999) Resection of colorectal liver metastases. Langenbecks Arch Surg 384:313–327
26. Semelka RC, Helmberger TK (2001) Contrast agents for MR imaging of the liver. Radiology 218:27–38
27. Semelka RC, Hussain SM, Marcos HB, Woosley JT (2000) Perilesional enhancement of hepatic metastases: correlation between MR imaging and histopathologic findings: initial observations. Radiology 215:89–94
28. Silverman SG, Tuncali K, Adams DF, vanSonnenberg E, Zou KH, Kacher DF, Morrison PR, Jolesz FA (2000) MR imaging-guided percutaneous cryotherapy of liver tumors: initial experience. Radiology 217:657–664
29. Stroszczynski C, Hosten N, Puls R, Nagel S, Scholman HJ, Wlodarczyk W, Oettle H, Moesta KT, Schlag PM, Felix R (2001) Histopathological correlation to MRI findings during and after laser-induced thermotherapy in a pig pancreas model. Invest Radiol 36:413–421
30. Stroszczynski C, Gretschel S, Gaffke G, Puls R, Kretzschmar A, Hosten N, Schlag PM, Felix R (2002) Laser-induced thermotherapy (LITT) for malignant liver tumours: the role of sonography in catheter placement and observation of the therapeutic procedure (in German). Ultraschall Med 23:163–167
31. Tranberg KG, Moller PH, Hannesson P, Stenram U (1994) Percutaneous interstitial laser hyperthermia in clinical use. Ann Chir Gynaecol 83:286–290
32. Veit P, Antoch G, Stergar H, Bockisch A, Forsting M, Kuehl H (2006) Detection of residual tumor after radiofrequency ablation of liver metastasis with dual-modality PET/CT: initial results. Eur Radiol 16:80–87
33. Vogl TJ, Muller PK, Hammerstingl R, Weinhold N, Mack MG, Philipp C, Deimling M, Beuthan J, Pegios W, Riess H et al. (1995) Malignant liver tumors treated with MR imaging-guided laser-induced thermotherapy: technique and prospective results. Radiology 196:257–265
34. Wlodarczyk W, Boroschewski R, Hentschel M, Wust P, Monich G, Felix R (1998) Three-dimensional monitoring of small temperature changes for therapeutic hyperthermia using MR. J Magn Reson Imaging 8:165–174

2 Development of Navigation Systems for Image-Guided Laparoscopic Tumor Resections in Liver Surgery

Thomas Lange, Michael Hünerbein, Sebastian Eulenstein,
Sigfried Beller, Peter Michael Schlag

Recent Results in Cancer Research, Vol. 167
© Springer-Verlag Berlin Heidelberg 2006

2.1 Introduction

Minimally invasive surgery has become a viable alternative to conventional surgery. The technical advantages of minimally invasive surgery can be translated into clinical benefits for the patients, i.e., less postoperative pain and impairment of lung function, better cosmetic results, shorter hospitalization, and earlier convalescence. Laparoscopic operations have replaced a significant proportion of open surgical procedures and are now routinely used. While the role of laparoscopic surgery has been generally accepted for the management of benign disorders, there is an ongoing debate regarding the adequacy of this technique in surgical oncology. There is evidence that minimally invasive surgery can reduce perioperative morbidity in cancer patients. However, definite validation of these procedures for tumor surgery is not yet available due to the lack of prospective randomized trials providing reliable long-term data on disease-free survival and overall survival. It seems likely that minimally invasive procedures will play an important role for the treatment of preneoplastic lesions and tumors of limited size.

There are some technical limitations to laparoscopic surgery. The degrees of freedom for the instruments are limited because of the minimal access via the trocars. The absence of direct organ palpation and the lack of the third dimension are still limits of laparoscopy. The surgeon's orientation and the location of anatomical and pathological structures is therefore more difficult than in open surgery. Modern image-guided surgery (IGS) systems have the potential to compensate these limitations. Preoperative computer-based intervention planning and intraoperative navigation systems are today routinely used for certain indications in neurosurgery, ENT and orthopedic surgery. Nevertheless major research efforts are still necessary to examine the clinical impact of image-guided surgery on current indications, to adapt the systems to other indications and to solve some open problems like intraoperative deformations.

In liver surgery, computer-assisted 3D modeling and planning based on preoperative CT or MRI data allows much more accurate planning of surgery and may help to select the optimal procedure [1]. Surgeons can obtain a better steric vision of the individual anatomy, the location of the tumor in relation to the vascular structures and the individual vascular territories defining the resection planes. The use of such planning systems in oncological surgery and liver transplantation is in routine use at some clinics and the number of users is increasing.

But at the end of this preparatory process, surgeons have to carry out the surgical plan on the patient in the OR. Intraoperative navigation systems support the surgeon to transfer preoperative plans precisely and safely. In neurosurgery, ENT surgery, orthopedic and trauma surgery navigation systems are well established for certain indications and several commercial systems are available. The main problem in liver surgery or in general in visceral surgery is the deformation of the liver or the organ of interest between preoperative imaging and the patient in the OR. Three-dimensional ultrasound is a promising intraoperative imaging modality to detect and solve this deformation problem.

In the following sections, the state of the art in computer-assisted liver surgery planning and the principles and technologies of conventional navigation systems in neurosurgery and orthopedic surgery is reviewed. Then the limitations of these navigation systems for soft tissue surgery are explained and current developments for open liver surgery are reported. Last, their transferability to laparoscopic procedures is discussed.

2.2 Computer-Assisted Liver Surgery Planning

2.2.1 Clinical Background

For surgery of malignant liver tumors, resection margins are important for long-term outcome [2]. Even though the width of surgical margins remains controversial [3–5], patients with a microscopically positive margin (R1) have a worse prognosis than R0-resected patients. It is the art of surgery to find a compromise between required radicality and optimal preservation of liver parenchyma.

Resections based on the extent of the tumor only (including a safety margin) are called atypical. Only in case of small tumors lying close beneath the liver surface should atypical resections be performed. In all other cases, the spatial relation of the tumor to the vascular system of the liver has to be taken into account (anatomical resection).

In contrast to many other organs, the liver possesses not only arteries and veins, but also a third blood vessel system, the portal veins. They drain venous blood from the entire gastrointestinal tract, thus supplying 80% of the liver's blood. For an anatomical resection, first vessel branches lying inside the safety margin as well as their dependent branches have to be identified. Next, the liver tissue supplied by these branches (called a vascular territory) has to be determined. Consequently, an entire section of the liver must be removed rather than the tumor on its own. Additionally, the drainage via the hepatic veins has to be ensured to avoid congestion.

Although today's imaging methods such as the multi-detector CT provide excellent visualization of the intrahepatic vascular system, neither the number and distribution nor the extent of liver territories can be determined distinctly. Hence, in oncological tumor resections, where the achievement of a certain safety margin may require the dissection of major intrahepatic vascular structures, areas at risk for devascularization can be identified only vaguely. Thus, prediction of the remaining and fully vascularized liver parenchyma is imprecise. Often only a coarse classification into eight segments after Couinaud is performed. But the vessel anatomy of individual patients varies greatly [6].

With the help of modern software tools the individual vascular territories can be computed based on a mathematical analysis of CT or MR data and the remaining vascularized liver parenchyma, depending on different resection planes, can be predicted. An important preliminary for these computations is a precise 3D modeling of the vascular system and parenchyma of the liver, as well as the tumor.

2.2.2 Three-Dimensional Modeling

The segmentation (extraction, labeling) of liver structures is the most challenging part of 3D modeling. Segmentation is the process in which each voxel (volume element) of the CT or MRI data is assigned (labeled) to a specific tissue: liver parenchyma, portal vein, tumor, etc. Based on this segmentation, it is standard to automatically generate tissue surfaces consisting of triangle meshes by the efficient marching cube algorithm [7]. For tube-like structures such as vessels, more sophisticated and specific surface-generation approaches such as truncated cones [8] and convolution surfaces [9] also exist, which provide smoother surfaces. Convolution surfaces even generate smooth surfaces at the branching of the vessels, as can be seen in Fig. 2.1.

Although Soler et al. [10] claimed a fully automatic segmentation procedure for the liver, they reported a 2-mm average deviation of liver parenchyma between manually and automatic segmentation evaluated on only five patients. Other institutions use manual or semi-automatic/interactive segmentation tools to segment the liver parenchyma [11]. At our institution, we currently also use semi-automatic tools (volume growing, intelligent scissors [12], shape-based interpolation [13]) to shorten the user interaction time. However, an automatic procedure is also under development, which will be described in the following.

The main problem for most general automatic or semi-automatic segmentation procedures is that at some locations the intensity contrast at the boundary of the liver is not sufficient or not given at all. The segmented liver tissue usually "leaks" into the surrounding tissue at those locations. One possibility to avoid such problems is to incorporate statistical knowledge about the anatomical shape of the liver into the segmentation process. The statistical model represents the average shape and the most important shape variations of a sample set of liver surfaces extracted from individual patients (Fig. 2.2). During the segmentation process, the statistical shape model is adapted to the individual liver shape by optimization of the model's parameters

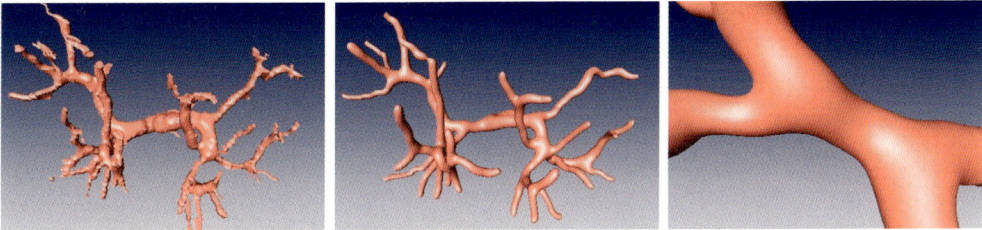

Fig. 2.1 Portal vein surface generated by marching cubes algorithm (*left*) and convolution surface method (*middle*). The convolution surface representation provides much smoother surfaces, even at branchings (*right*)

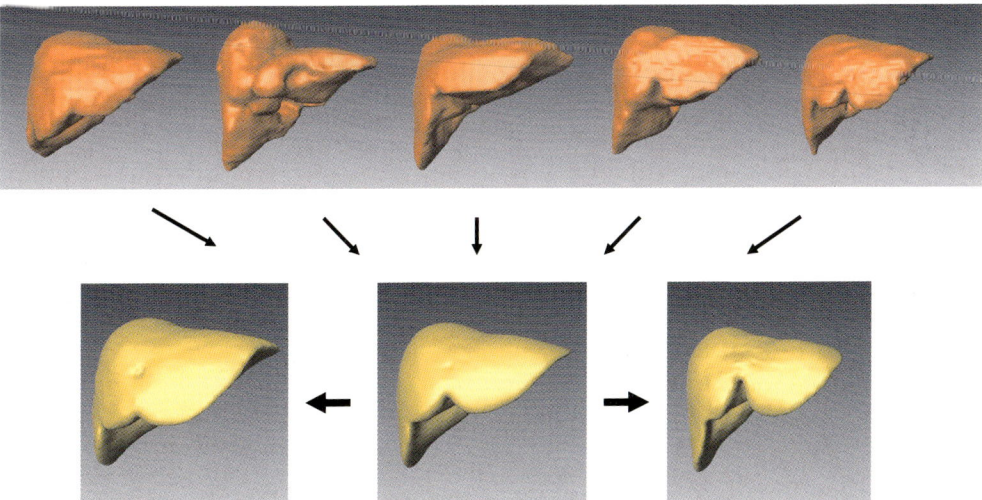

Fig. 2.2 Liver surfaces of 43 individual patients (*top row*) are assembled to a parameterized statistical shape model (*bottom row*) for automatic liver segmentation. The mean liver shape (*middle*) and the range of the parameter representing the first main shape variation are shown (*left and right*)

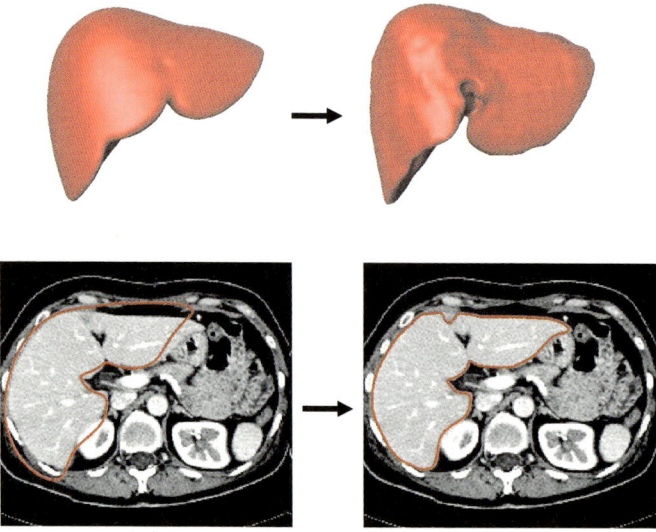

Fig. 2.3 The average liver shape is rigidly fitted to the individual patient (*left*) and then the parameters of the shape model are optimized to recover the individual shape (*right*)

(Fig. 2.3). Hence those models are also called active shape models (ASMs) [14]. The optimization criterion is based on intensity values along lines perpendicular to the surface of the liver. We built a shape model of the liver from 43 patients [15] and investigated the performance of the approach for 33 contrast-enhanced CT scans [16, 17]. An average accuracy of 2.3 (±0.3) mm of surface distance was achieved. Although not fully satisfactory until now, the approach is promising, because an improvement in the accuracy with an increasing number of sample shapes in the model can be observed. Thus further improvements might be achieved by extending the model.

In most cases, the segmentation of vessels is easier than parenchyma segmentation because the contrast is higher as a result of contrast agent injection. However, another problem exists when building precise models containing portal veins as well as hepatic veins. In contrast-enhanced bi- or tri-phase imaging, two or three acquisitions are carried out at different points in time depending on the arrival time of the contrast agent in arteries and portal and hepatic veins. First, the contrast agent reaches the arteries (arterial phase), then the portal veins (portal venous phase), and last the hepatic veins (hepatic venous phase). In the portal venous (PV) phase, the hepatic veins are not enhanced. However, in the hepatic venous (HV) phase, portal veins are typically also visible, but with lower contrast than in the portal venous phase. To derive high-quality vessel models, portal veins should be segmented from a PV phase and hepatic veins from a HV phase (Fig. 2.4). PV as well as HV images are acquired during respiration hold, which is normally at end-inspiration. Unfortunately, if the patient breathes between the acquisitions – the position and shape of the liver cannot be reproduced exactly. Consequently, if segmentations of portal and hepatic veins from different phases are used in a single model, the phases must be registered. Registration is the process of determining a geometrical transformation that maps each point in one data set (model) to its anatomically corresponding point in the other data set (reference).

We investigated to what extent the liver's position and shape changes between the portal venous and the hepatic venous phases, and whether these changes can be eliminated by rigid, and if necessary, by non-rigid mutual information based on automatic registration. Mutual information is a commonly used distance measure for intensity images. The investigations cover CT as well as MRI data. The study showed that in most cases, patients are not able to reproduce

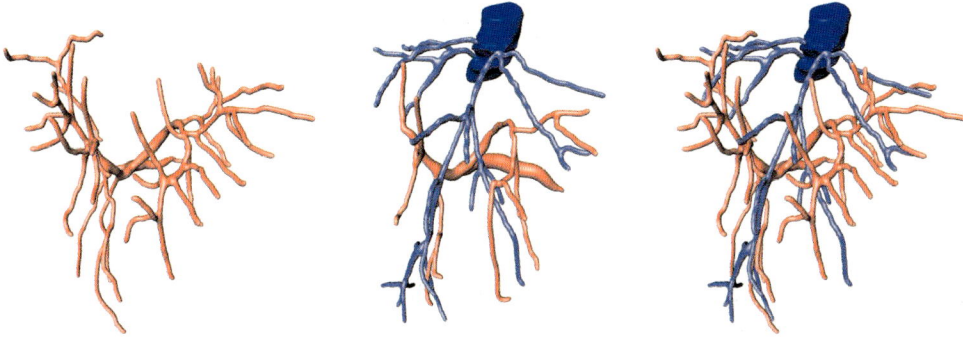

Fig. 2.4 Portal (*pink*) and hepatic (*blue*) veins are displayed in the portal venous (PV) (*left*) and hepatic venous (HV) phase (*middle*). A combination of portal veins from the PV and hepatic veins from the HV phase is visualized in the right image

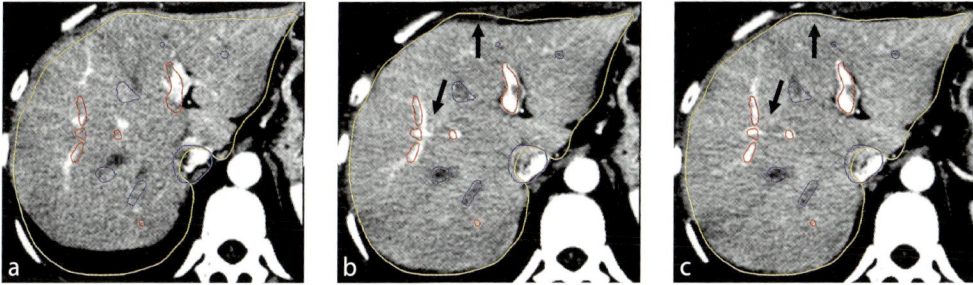

Fig. 2.5a–c Portal venous phase (underlying image) and hepatic venous phase (overlaid intersections) do not match because of different respiratory states (**a**). Rigid (**b**) and in particular nonrigid (**c**) registration compensates the mismatch

the respiratory state of PV phase in the HV phase exactly (7.2±4.2 mm movement on average) and at least rigid registration is necessary [18]. However, only in some cases is non-rigid registration needed to compensate significant deformations in the range of 2–3 mm (Fig. 2.5).

2.2.3 Features of Planning Systems

Several systems have been developed for liver surgery planning in the last few years based on 3D models generated from CT or MRI data [10, 19, 20]. There is even a commercial service that offers processing of CT/MRI data for liver surgery planning (MeVis Distant Services AG, Bremen, Germany). These systems are applied for planning living donor liver transplantations (LDLTs) [21, 22] and oncological liver resections for individual patient anatomies [23–25]. In LDLTs, the liver must be split into in a well-preserved graft and a remnant liver lobe without damaging the donor. The aim in oncological liver surgery is to remove the tumor completely while conserving as much healthy tissue as possible.

The visualization of a virtual 3D model of the liver is a valuable tool for the surgeon to better imagine the individual vessel anatomy and in oncological liver surgery the spatial relation of a tumor to these vessels. The distance of the tumor to the surrounding vessels can also be quantified. Anatomical variants such as trifurcation of the portal vein or aberrant or accessory hepatic arteries are a common finding and can be appropriately visualized by the surgeon.

For LDLTs as well as for oncological resections, it is important to know exactly the individual vascular territories, as explained in Sect. 2.1. A vascular territory represents a part of the liver that is supplied or drained by a certain vascular branch. The idea of computer-based vascular territory determination is that the closer a parenchyma voxel is to a vascular branch, the more likely is it for this voxel to be supplied by the branch [19]. Although only a coarse approximation of the underlying physiology, good estimations are obtained. Besides the portovenous supply, the venous outflow of a vascular territory is also computed [22, 25, 26] (see Fig. 2.6). With modern multidetector scanners, even hepatic arteries and bile ducts can be incorporated [22].

Based on the vascular territories an automatic risk analysis of blood supply and drainage can be performed according to the location of a tumor or an interactively defined resection plane. By interactively changing the resection plane, the impact of different surgical strategies on the arterial devascularization and venous congestion volumes can be predicted. Lang et al. [26] state that computer-assisted risk analysis can influence the operation plan of liver resections compared to standard 2D CT. The consistency of the computed virtual vascular territories and real territories has only been evaluated on corrosion casts so far [19]. An evaluation for the liver in vivo is an important task for further research.

2.3 Principles, Technologies, and Conventional Implementations of Navigation Systems

Three-dimensional liver resection planning supports the surgeon in many cases and is routinely used in some institutions, although there is no clear indication which patients truly need such planning and to what extent. The most important problem is how to transfer this plan to the patient in the OR. Until now, the results of preoperative planning (3D anatomical model, definition of resection volumes, etc.) had to be mentally transferred by the surgeon to the patient in the operating room (OR). There is no navigation system to help the surgeon precisely localize the tumor, major vessels, and vascular territories during liver surgery. Several commercial 3D navigation systems for image-guided surgery are available for bony structures, e.g., in neurosurgery or orthopedics, but there are only few systems – mostly research systems – that deal with navigation in soft tissue, as is the case

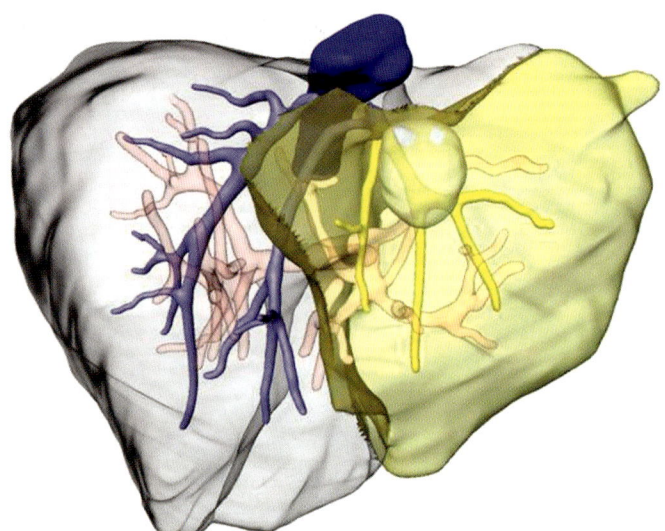

Fig. 2.6 An example of preoperative liver resection planning. The left hepatic vein (*yellow*) has to be cut through because of the close location to the tumor. The part of the liver tissue (vascular territory) that is drained by the left hepatic vein is marked yellow. This part is at risk for congestions if not resected

in liver surgery. The reason for this is that bony structures do not change their shape between preoperative acquisition of image data such as MRI or CT scans and positioning the patient for surgery. Thus, it is possible to register preoperative images rigidly to the physical patient space. In liver surgery, the liver usually deforms significantly between preoperative imaging and positioning the patient in the OR.

Before approaches for liver navigation systems are explained, a short review on principles and technologies of conventional navigation systems used in neurosurgery and orthopedic surgery is given.

2.3.1 Principles of Conventional Navigation Systems

The concept of a navigation system, for example in neurosurgery, is to use images of the brain to guide the surgeon to a target within the brain. The spatial relation of a surgical instrument to the location of anatomical and pathological structures is visualized on a monitor. It is possible to look inside the patient. An image-guided navigation system consists of a pre- or intraoperative imaging modality, a tracking or position sensing system to track the location of an instrument, and a computer as well as a software for control and visualization.

Two important aspects of a navigation system are the intraoperative registration of the image data and the calibration of instruments and possibly intraoperative imaging devices. Registration and calibration are also main factors influencing the accuracy of a navigation system. Because images (CT or MRI) are often acquired preoperatively, the image space and the real world coordinate system of the patient in the OR have to be spatially related. In most cases, a rigid transformation (TR) based on bony structures or artificial markers is determined. An example using

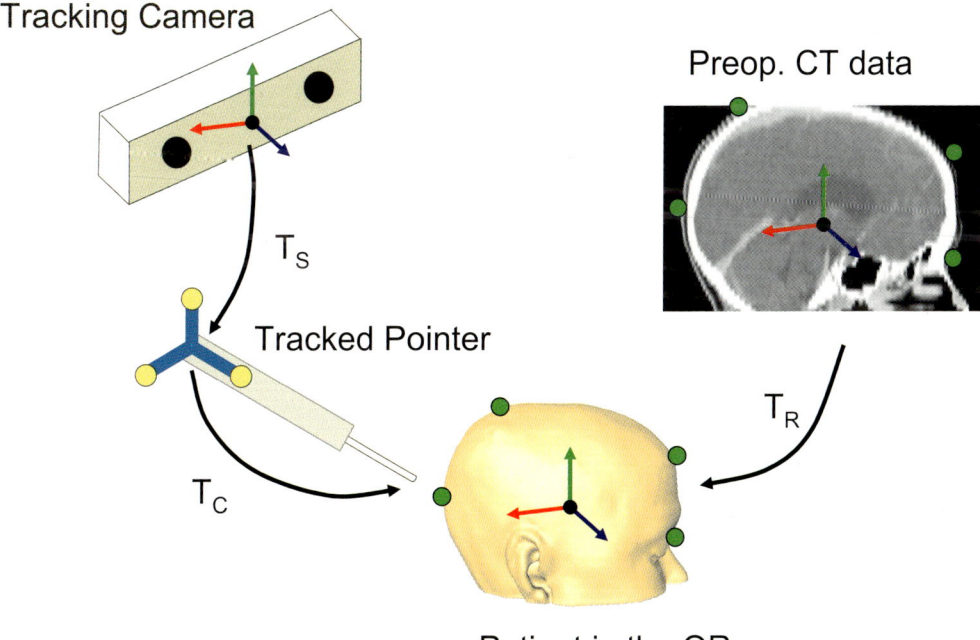

Fig. 2.7 Principle of conventional navigation system based on preoperative CT data and image-to-patient registration via landmarks identified by a tracked pointer

markers is illustrated in Fig. 2.7. A more detailed description of different registration concepts is given in Sect. 3.3.

In a calibration process, rigid transformations (TC) are computed to map local coordinate systems of instruments or intraoperative imaging devices to coordinate systems of the tracking system sensors. Before calibration is explained in more detail, the mode of operation of different tracking technologies is described.

2.3.2 Tracking Systems

The heart of a navigation system is a tracking system. Those systems are also called position-sensing systems or localizer systems. A tracking system consists of one or several sensors attached to a surgical instrument or an ultrasound probe that are tracked by a device calculating the position and orientation of the sensors. There are four different technologies to track medical instruments: mechanical, acoustical, electromagnetic, and optical.

2.3.2.1 Mechanical

A mechanical localizer is an articulated arm whose tip position can be determined by the angles of the joints. An example of this technology is the FARO surgical arm (FARO Medical Technologies, Orlando, FL, USA). Mechanical arms are very accurate, but can only track one object at a time and are cumbersome. Therefore they are rarely used in surgery nowadays.

2.3.2.2 Acoustical

The general idea of acoustical tracking systems is that US waves are emitted by speakers and received by microphones. By measuring either the propagation time or phase differences, positions can be determined. Because the accuracy of these systems is affected by variations in pressure, temperature, and humidity, they are also used only in a few medical applications. In addition, a free line of sight between speakers and microphones is mandatory.

2.3.2.3 Electromagnetic

A magnetic field is generated by a transmitter (field generator). The induced electrical current in a coil (sensor) is measured. Because the distribution of the magnetic field is known, the position and orientation of the sensor can be computed. The magnetic field is either generated by alternating current (AC) or directed current (DC). AC as well as DC devices are sensitive to some types of metals in their surroundings and to magnetic fields generated, for example, by power generators or monitors. Both technologies are affected by ferromagnetic materials (e.g., iron, steel), because they change the homogeneity of the generated magnetic field. AC technology is more affected by good conductors such as copper and aluminum because of distortions caused by eddy currents. Examples of AC electromagnetic tracking devices are the Polhemus models (Polhemus Inc., Colchester, VT, USA), for DC devices the models of Ascension (Ascension Technologies, Burlington, VT, USA) and NDI (Northern Digital Inc., Waterloo, ON, Canada). The advantage of electromagnetic tracking systems for clinical use is that no free line of sight between sensors and field generator has to be ensured. Thus it is possible to track very small sensor coils inserted in needles or catheters in the interior of the body. To date, only a few navigation systems use electromagnetic tracking devices (e.g., Medtronic StealthStation AXIEM, Minneapolis, MN, USA, GE InstaTrack, and ENTrack, Milwaukee, WI, USA) because of the inaccuracies induced by metals in the operating field. But the new generation of electromagnetic tracking systems (NDI Aurora, Medtronic StealthStation AXIEM) has significantly improved [27]. The accuracy of electromagnetic tracking systems is a around 1 mm.

2.3.2.4 Optical

The principle of optical tracking is to locate the position of optical markers with multiple cameras. Because the optical markers are detected from at least two cameras with a known spatial relation to each other, the 3D position of the markers can be computed by triangulation. At least three of these markers are mounted on a rigid frame (tracker), so that the orientation of the tracker can be determined. Additional markers increase visibility and measurement accuracy. Different geometrical configurations of the markers on the trackers allow the trackers to be distinguished. The markers can be infrared light-emitting diodes (active markers, passive infrared-sensitive camera), infrared light-reflecting spheres (passive markers, active infrared-emitting and infrared-sensitive camera), or high-contrast targets (passive cameras, passive markers).

Today, most surgical navigation systems use optical tracking devices, because of their high accuracy and reliability. The accuracy of the typically used Polaris two camera system (NDI) is 0.35 mm RMS (root mean square) measured at 500 different positions of the measurement volume. The only significant disadvantage of optical systems compared to electromagnetic devices in some applications is the free line of sight issue.

2.3.2.5 Calibration of Tracker

To understand the functionality of a navigation system, it is important to understand that a tracking system determines the position and orientation of the sensors mounted on the surgical instruments or ultrasound transducer, but not directly the location of the instrument's tip or the image coordinate system of the ultra sound transducer. Because the sensor is fixed on the instrument, a rigid transformation (TC) from the sensor to the instrument tip can be determined (see Fig. 2.7). This process is called calibration. Instruments can be calibrated before surgery, if the sensors are already mounted on the instrument, or can be reproducible attached to the instrument. Another possibility is to calibrate the instruments in the operating room by means of calibration blocks. Calibration of surgical instruments is quiet easy, but calibration of an ultrasound device is more complicated and time-consuming, such that it is usually done preoperatively.

2.3.3 Intraoperative Patient-to-Image Registration

The general idea of patient-to-image registration methods is to identify points or surfaces usually on bony structures that can be identified precisely in the preoperative image data as well as intraoperatively in the physical patient. In conventional systems, only rigid transformations are determined to relate preoperative image space and the real-world coordinate system of the patient.

2.3.3.1 Stereotactic Frame

Image-guided surgery has its roots in the field of stereotaxy and stereotactic surgery [28]. The stereotactic frame is mounted at the patient's head to provide a rigid reference that establishes a coordinate system relative to the patient, to supply recognizable landmarks in the images, and provide a stable mounting and guide for instruments used to perform the neurosurgical procedures. The stereotactic frame forms the gold standard of reference systems for image-guided surgery. A similar, but noninvasive approach is to use a headset that can be reproducibly mounted on the patient and is also worn during imaging and surgery [29].

2.3.3.2 Landmarks

Another noninvasive method is to use landmarks. The general idea of artificial (fiducial) or anatomical landmarks is to define points in the image data that can be identified with a tracked pointer in the OR. The landmark registration process is also called point matching. One possibility is to define anatomical landmarks such as the nasion and the tragus of the ears in neurosurgery. This approach is not fully satisfactory, because there is some variation in the identified locations of the landmark points on the patient, as well as a problem of identifying exactly the same locations within the patient's image data. The accuracy and precision can be improved somewhat by using surface markers glued to the patient's skin. Their location can be more precisely determined by the pointer, and they can be automatically identified in the image data. But due to skin movements with respect to the underlying bony structures, inaccuracies can occur. Maurer et al. [30] have demonstrated that the only way to achieve patient-to-image registration with the same accuracy as can be obtained with a stereotactic frame is using bone-mounted fiducial markers. But like the stereotactic frame, the implantation of the bone markers is also invasive.

2.3.3.3 Surface Registration

All of the above-mentioned registration methods are either invasive or special markers or headsets have to be attached to the patient already during imaging. This often requires more imaging in addition to previous diagnostic imaging. Anatomical landmarks are noninvasive and markerless, but accuracy is not satisfactory. Surface registration methods have the potential to increase accuracy while being noninvasive and easy to use.

In contrast to landmark registration, arbitrary points on a surface such as the face are intraoperatively acquired. These surface points are then matched with the corresponding surface in the preoperative image data by means of the iterative closest point (ICP) algorithm [31]. Different possibilities exist for the intraoperative acquisition of the surface points. The easiest method is to use a tracked pointer. More convenient and contactless are laser scanning methods. With handheld systems such as the z-touch from BrainLAB (Heimstätten, Germany) [32], approximately 100 surface points are acquired by manual movement. The z-touch projects an infrared point onto the patient's face. This infrared spot is identified with the infrared tracking camera of the navigation system. In a few seconds, a laser range scanner measures the entire surface at once with up to some 100 000 points. Because of the high number of scanned surface points, very accurate registration results can be achieved [33]. Nevertheless, one has to be aware that skin movements significantly degrade the accuracy.

All conventional image-guided surgery systems operate on the assumption that the tissue being operated on can be treated as a rigid body that does not change its form between the time the preoperative images are acquired and the surgery is performed. But even in neurosurgery this assumption does not hold, as the so-called brain-shift problem illustrates. This problem will be discussed in more detail in Sect. 4 and possible solutions will be shown.

2.3.4 Intraoperative Visualization

If the patient has been registered in the OR and all instruments are calibrated the spatial relation and movement of surgical instruments to a target region (for example, a tumor) and adjacent organs at risk are visualized in real time on a monitor. Because only a 2D projection of anatomical structures can be shown on the monitor, different visualization techniques have been developed to guide the surgeon in 3D space. A standard technique is to show several 2D slices (section planes) of the preoperative CT or MRI acquisition (multiplanar image display). These slices are often perpendicular to each other and are chosen and updated according to the location of a surgical instrument. Sometimes slices also are used that are perpendicular to the instrument axis, showing a view in the direction of the instrument. Particularly in neurosurgery, multimodal image display can increase the information level by showing registered preoperative CT and MRI data together.

Often additionally or in orthopedics, 3D surface models (surface shading) are also shown to give a better overview. This surface modeling first requires an easy delineation of the relevant structures, which is often automatically only possible for bony structures. An alternative is to visualize anatomical structures by direct volume rendering. No explicit segmentation or surface extraction is necessary. Volume rendering employs a ray-tracing technique where image values along the rays are integrated according to a transfer function. With suitable transfer functions, some anatomical structures can be excellently visualized in real-time.

In principle, stereoscopic 3D displays may improve depth perception, but to date they have not prevailed in clinical routine.

A promising approach for intraoperative visualization is augmented reality [34]. In augmented reality, real views and virtual models are merged to one common augmented visualization. One example for augmented reality visualization that is in clinical use in neuronavigation is the contour-guided approach provided by the MKM microscope (Zeiss, Oberkochen, Germany) [35]. In the microscopic field through the eyepieces, the surgeon sees virtual contours of the patient's brain tumor superimposed on the actual tumor. The projected contours correspond to the current focus plane of the microscope.

In addition to this established approach, other augmented reality methods are an active field of research. Augmented reality is divided into head-mounted displays (HMDs) and monitor- or screen-based methods on the one hand and into video see-through and optical see-through devices on the other hand. In an early study, State et al. [36] presented a stereoscopic video see-through HMD for ultrasound-guided biopsies. The advantage of an HMD is that the virtual models are exactly projected into the view direction of the surgeon, because the position of the HMD is tracked. For medical purposes, optical see-throughs might be more appropriate, but generally the ergonomics of HMD technologies needs to be improved to be accepted by surgeons. The acceptance of monitor- or screen-based techniques is possibly greater. Grimson et al. [37] demonstrated a monitor-based video see-through approach on a neurosurgical example. One example for a screen-based optical see-through technique was introduced by Fichtinger et al. [38] for the purpose of percutaneous CT-guided needle interventions. This optical-see through technique is implemented by mounting a half mirror and a flat panel LCD display on the gantry of the CT scanner. The surgeon looks trough the half mirror and sees an overlay of the LCD monitor. An alternative technique is a transparent LCD display [39]. One interesting approach that does not fit into the previous classification is projector-based augmented reality, where virtual models are directly projected onto the patient anatomy [40].

2.4 Soft Tissue Navigation Based on Preoperative Image Data

The main challenge in the development of navigation systems for soft tissue surgery is to solve the problem of tissue deformations. All conventional image-guided surgery systems operate on the assumption that the tissue being operated on can be treated as a rigid body that does not change its form between the time the preoperative images are acquired and the surgery is performed. Even in neurosurgery, the accuracy of navigation systems is decreased by deformations of the brain after opening the dura: the so called brain-shift. In principle, two different approaches are possible to solve the deformation issue: the use of an intraoperative imaging modality to obtain an up-to-date image in the OR or to measure points or surfaces of anatomical structures directly in the OR and perform a nonrigid registration algorithm to compensate for the deformations. Until now, only first attempts have been made regarding approaches without intraoperative imaging.

2.4.1 Landmark-Based Approaches

Some groups are trying to transfer the conventional navigation approach based on landmarks and rigid registration to soft tissue surgery, in particular to laparoscopic surgery. For some regions in the abdomen, this might be possible with limited accuracy. Mårvik et al. [41] investigated the landmark-based registration accuracy for laparoscopic adrenalectomies on six patients. Skin markers were glued to the patient prior to MRI/CT scanning and images were acquired with the patient in the same position as projected for the OR. The registration was performed by placing a pointer intraoperatively into the markers before insufflation. Than a rigid laparoscopic navigation pointer (LNP) helped the surgeon to identify locations of organs, tumors, and vessels. An average patient registration accuracy of 6.9 mm FRE (fiducial registration error) was achieved, because the insufflation did not cause anatomic shifts in the retroperitoneum. The use of the LNP for anatomical structures in the anterior part of the abdomen was excluded due to significantly higher anatomic shift. It was proposed to use intraoperative 3D ultrasound to compensate for this shift, as was suggested in a feasibility study conducted by Kaspersen et al. [42] for navigated stent-graft implantation of abdominal aortic aneurysms. The study was based on transcutaneous ultrasound, and a mismatch of 13 mm (4.6–23.1 mm) on average in 33 patients was reported between ultrasound and registered CT imaging at the aorta. The mismatch was quantified by manual registration of ultrasound and CT images. It has to be taken into account that the aorta is fairly rigidly attached to the spine, and therefore does not move much with respiration, which occurs, for example, for the liver.

Landmark-based registration was also used for navigated percutaneous CT-guided liver punctures [43]. One aim was to enable out-of-plane needle guidance for radio frequency (RF) ablations or biopsies [44]. Nicolau et al. [45] developed a video-based augmented reality system for liver punctures that automatically identifies skin markers in video images and performs a 3D/2D registration in real time. They achieved an average accuracy of 9.5 mm on three patients [46] compared to 8.3 mm in swine experiments reported by Banovac et al. [43]. In both studies, the CT was acquired immediately before the puncture. However, [43] the swine had to be transported from the CT scanner to the angiography suite, possibly introducing change in the animal's position. While Nicolau et al. conducted their experiments under free patient breathing, Banovac et al. tried to minimize the error introduced by respiratory motion by obtaining the preprocedural CT scan in full expiration, and performing their registration in the angiography suite in full expiration as well.

2.4.2 Surface-Based Approaches

Two approaches for surface registration of preoperative CT scans of the liver to physical patient space have been reported in the literature. Herline et al. [47] digitized the liver surface by moving an optically tracked probe over the visible portions of a liver phantom and rigidly registering it to the liver surface extracted from CT scans by the iterative closest point (ICP) algorithm. A contactless variant of this approach has been implemented by Cash et al. [48] using a commercial laser range scanner instead of a tracked probe. They performed phantom studies and have applied their system to one clinical case so far. A mean residual error of 1.72±1.43 mm for the clinical case and target registration errors (TREs) ranging from 0.6 mm to 7.74 mm for different tumors embedded in a deformable phantom were reported. Nevertheless, it is not clear how accurately tumors lying deep inside the liver are registered in clinical cases. An improved version has been published by Sinha et al. [49] incorporating texture information. Sun et al. [50] recently introduced an alternative elegant contactless approach to measure the cortical surface by means of a stereoscopic operating microscope. The 3D surface is estimated from a stereo pair of images from the microscope. They report measured motion of the cortical surface during ten clinical cases. They suggest using the captured cortical displacement data to aid computational biomechanical brain models to estimate deformations of the whole brain volume, in particular in the depth of the brain.

2.4.3 Model-Updated Image-Guided Surgery

The assumption that the brain and in particular the liver is rigid has been shown not to hold true in many cases, and significant soft tissue deformation is often present. Several groups have developed biomechanical models of soft tissue mainly for the brain [51], but also for the liver [52]. The development of precise physically based models is challenging because of how difficult it is to quantify in vivo tissue behavior and the need for sophisticated and time-efficient mathematical methods such as the finite element method (FEM). It is important to note that different qualitative models are used. Often the tissue behavior is simplified by assuming linear elastic materials [53], which does hold only for small deformations. For higher strains, the stress–strain relationship for soft tissues is nonlinear [54, 55]. The tissue parameters differ between different patients. Quantitative MRI or ultrasound elastography might enable measurement of these individual parameters.

The idea of model-updated image-guided surgery is to measure intraoperatively sparse data that drive and constrain patient-specific biomechanical models. The aim is to adapt those preoperative models to the intraoperative situs. These intraoperative data can be captured surface displacements [56–58], as described in the previous section, or as will be discussed in the next sections, subsurface displacements captured by, for example, intraoperative ultrasound [59].

2.5 Navigation for Open Liver Surgery Based on Intraoperative Imaging

The application of intraoperative imaging modalities offers the possibility to obtain up-to-date information of the location and shape of an organ of interest in the OR. In neurosurgery, intraoperative 1.5-T high-field MR scanners have been integrated into the OR [60, 61] and have been combined with navigation systems. Whole integrated operating rooms are offered commercially (BrainSuite from BrainLab). CT scanners are rarely used intraoperatively, but are often used for image-guided interventions. Instead, mobile fluoroscopic devices (C-arms) have been an integral part of the standard equipment used in orthopedic and trauma surgery for quite some time. C-arm-based navigation systems can, for example, improve the accuracy of pedicle screw insertion [62]. A promising advancement is navigation systems based on 3D C-arm fluoroscopy, also called 3D rotational X-ray imaging (3DRX) [62, 63].

Ultrasound is an intraoperative imaging modality that is inexpensive compared to intraoperative MRI, and radiation-free, unlike fluoroscopy. In addition, ultrasound can easily be integrated into the OR. Navigated 2D ultrasound (Sononavigation) is a valuable tool for detecting brain-shift [64, 65]. In some neuronavigation systems, real-time 2D ultrasound has been integrated just recently, e.g., IGsonic from Brainlab or SonoNav from Medtronic.

In open and in particular laparoscopic liver surgery, intraoperative 2D ultrasound (IOUS) is routinely used. However, navigated 2D ultrasound has only been reported once for liver punctures [66].

Sononavigation based on 3D ultrasound is a consequent advancement and improvement. Until now only a few manufacturers have offered 3D ultrasound devices and only a single commercial navigation system based on 3D ultrasound exists (SonoWand from MISON, Trondheim, Norway). But before 3D ultrasound navigation is explained in more detail, existing 3D ultrasound technologies are introduced.

2.5.1 Three-Dimensional Ultrasound Technologies

Four different 3D ultrasound technologies exist.

1. 3D ultrasound probes consisting of 2D arrays
2. 3D probes mechanically or electronically steered
3. 2D tracked probe or freehand
4. Sensorless techniques

Sensorless tracking is done by analyzing the speckle in the US images using decorrelation [67] or linear regression [68]. Encouraging results have presented, but practical performance of in vivo imaging has to be further evaluated. In freehand 3D ultrasound, a position sensor of a localizer system is clamped to a conventional 2D US transducer and the transducer is manually swept over the volume of interest while the position and orientation of the imaging planes are recorded by the localizer system. After scanning, the 2D image planes are composed into a 3D image volume. In contrast to freehand 3D ultrasound, mechanically steered 3D probes do not rely on tracking sensors. Instead, a 2D transducer is swept by a motor contained in a specific 3D ultrasound probe. One example of such a system using a motor is the VOLUSON system developed by Kretztechnik and now distributed by General Electric (Milwaukee, WI, USA). A promising and just recently commercially available alternative is volumetric 3D probes containing a 2D array of transducer elements, such that 3D volumes can be directly measured.

Generally, all 3D ultrasound technologies are suitable as a basis for intraoperative navigation systems. We prefer mechanically steered 3D probes, because they are very easy to manage in the OR. The 3D transducer is held directly onto the liver in open surgery for only a few seconds, depending on the image resolution and scan angles.

2.5.2 Navigation Systems Based on 3D Ultrasound

The general principle of a 3D ultrasound-based navigation system is similar to that of a conventional neuronavigation system regarding instrument tracking and visualization. The difference is the use of intraoperative instead of preoperative image data and the kind of registration to relate image space and physical patient space. No explicit registration is necessary. A position sensor is attached to the ultrasound probe and the location of the probe during acquisition is measured (T_{S2}). If in addition the position and orientation of the ultrasound image coordinate system is known in relation to the location of the position sensor on the probe (T_{C2}), the spatial relationship between image space and physical patient space is also determined (see Fig. 2.8). The process of computing the transformation (T_{C2}) that converts the ultrasound image space into the coordinate system of the position sensor attached to the probe is called calibration. As calibration is a time-consuming process that must be performed very precisely, it is usually performed once and a suitable mounting ensures a reproducible attachment of the position sensor. A comprehensive overview of calibration techniques is given by Mercier et al. [69].

To our knowledge, only one 3D ultrasound navigation system is commercially available: SonoWand [70] from MISON. This system was developed for neurosurgery and experiences on brain tumor resections of 91 patients were reported [71]. SonoWand is based on freehand 3D US and the optical tracking system Polaris (NDI, Radolfzell, Germany). Lindseth et al. [72] have extensively investigated the laboratory accuracy of the system and found a mean deviation of 1.40±0.45 mm. Improper probe calibration was the main contributor to this error. Display techniques may be conventional orthogonal slices oriented to the patient (axial, sagittal, coronal), from the surgeon's view, or only defined by the position and orientation of the surgical tool. In any plane slicing, only one slice defined by the

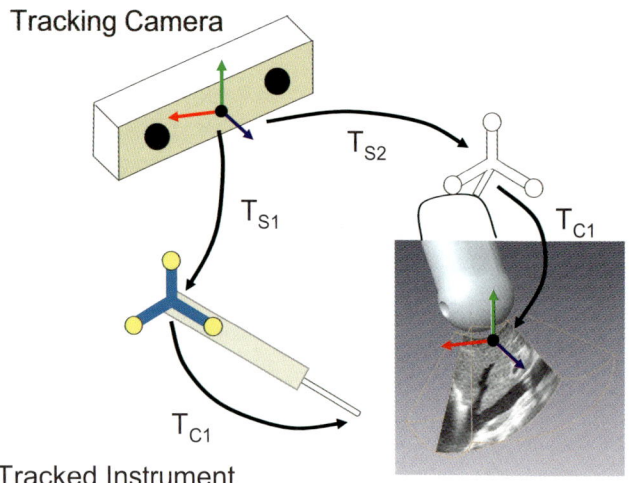

Fig. 2.8 Principle of a navigation system based on intraoperative 3D ultrasound using a tracked 3D probe

position and orientation of the surgical tool is displayed from each 3D volume. Another 3D update (ultrasound acquisition) was acquired whenever tissue changes made it unsafe to proceed; typically, updates were obtained three to six times during a surgical procedure.

At our clinic, we have developed a 3D ultrasound navigation system dedicated to oncological liver resections. Until now, the system has been in clinical use for open surgery, but can be extended for laparoscopic surgery as well. The general principle is similar to the SonoWand system, but the main difference is the motor-driven 3D ultrasound technology used (Voluson 730 Kretztechnik/GE) and the possibility of computer-assisted liver resection planning based on preoperative CT/MRI data. The 3D probe has been calibrated in a laboratory setting with a commercial 3D ultrasound phantom (CIRS, model 055) containing two egg-shaped structures.

The clinical procedure is as follows. Preoperatively, a computer-assisted plan of the liver resection is performed, as described in Sect. 2. The configuration of the navigation system in the OR is outlined in Fig. 2.9. The surgical procedure starts with mobilization and exposure of the liver. The 3D ultrasound probe is put into a sterile drape and a sterile position sensor is attached to the ultrasound probe. Before the actual resection, a 3D ultrasound scan consisting of simultaneous B-mode and power Doppler (PD) acquisition is performed in a few seconds. The location of the attached passive position sensor is measured during the acquisition by a Polaris tracking system. The data are digitally transferred in high quality and original resolution to the navigation system via a DICOM interface and not via the video output. Then a tracked electrocautery device can be navigated in relation to the 3D ultrasound data.

Two section planes of the ultrasound data are visualized (see Fig. 2.10). One plane is in line with the ultrasound probe and one perpendicular representing a view in the direction of the probe. The probe is in general oriented on the liver surface such that the first plane is an approximately sagittal slice and the other an approximately coronal slice. Tumor borders as well as vessels can be identified on these planes. The power Doppler data are overlaid on the B-mode data. Structures are projected onto the liver surface and mapped with the tracked electrocautery device used as a pointer and marker. This requires the position of the coronal plane to be frozen at the level of greatest interest. To map the tumor borders, this plane is set into the largest diameter of the tumor (Fig. 2.10a). To map vessels, the plane can also be moved and tilt into the longitudinal axis of the

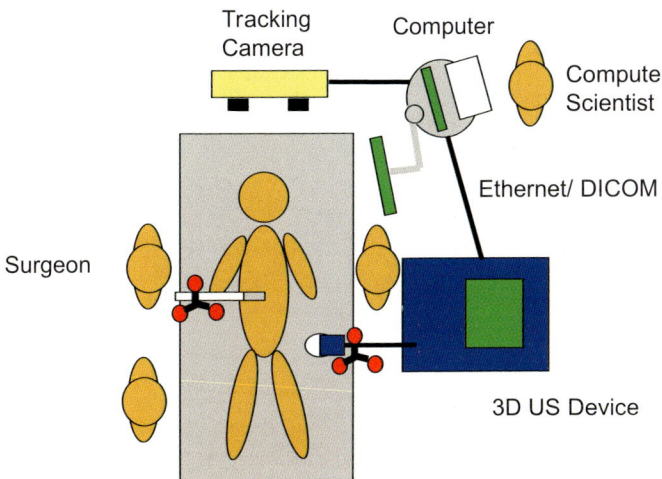

Fig. 2.9 Configuration of the 3D ultrasound-based navigation system in the OR

vessel (Fig. 2.10b). Tumor borders and relevant vessels in the tumor area are branded with blue and red ink onto the liver surface.

A first feasibility study on 30 patients showed that the system supports the surgeon in exactly carrying out the preoperative surgical plan intraoperatively. The system can be easily integrated into the OR and worked robustly. The additional operation time for navigation was acceptable. A detailed description of the study will be published elsewhere. The clinical accuracy of the system depends on deformations possibly induced by the transducer pressure, respiration, and heart movement. These factors must be quantified in future work.

One limitation of the current procedure is that during the actual resection, no navigation is performed. Repetitive ultrasound acquisitions are conceivable, but if a Pringle maneuver is conducted vessels are difficult to identify. A second limitation is that the preoperative plan is mentally transferred to the ultrasound data. Therefore work in progress on automatic transfer of preoperative models on the patient in the OR is presented.

2.5.3 Augmentation of Intraoperative Ultrasound with Preoperative Models

Three-dimensional ultrasound is well suited for liver surgery navigation, because vessels have good contrast, particularly in power Doppler ultrasound. However, tumors are sometimes difficulty to delineate. Transmission of portal vein, hepatic vein, tumor, and liver surface models from preoperative CT/MR scans onto ultrasound images can significantly improve differentiation of these structures. The relation of ultrasound planes to preoperative data or models would increase the orientation ability of the surgeon. In addition, the transmission of a preoperative resection plan to the patient in the OR would be possible.

For the transmission of the preoperative data onto the US images, a registration algorithm is needed. This algorithm has to be fast and robust and must be able to compensate significant deformations. There are only a few studies published regarding automatic rigid or nonrigid registration methods that have been applied or adapted to 3D ultrasound data. Some image-based methods [73–75] have been reported to rigidly register 3D ultrasound and MRI data.

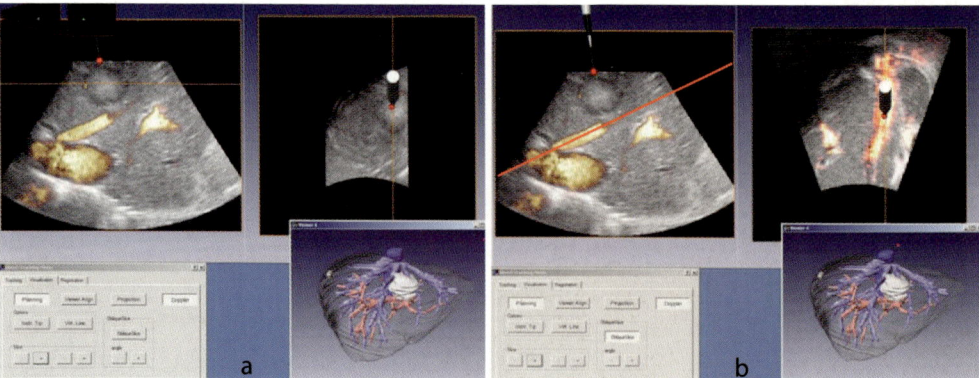

Fig. 2.10a,b Intraoperative visualization by two section planes of the ultrasound data. Power Doppler information is overlaid on the B-mode data. Additionally the preoperative planning model is shown. In **a** the coronal slice (*right*) is orthogonal to the sagittal slice. In **b** the orientation of the coronal slice is adapted to the direction of a hepatic vein close to the tumor

Nonrigid image-based algorithms for registration of two ultrasound volumes are described in [75, 76]. These approaches are usually too time-consuming for intraoperative use. A reduction of the image content to significant features might accelerate the procedure. Liver vessels are features that can be easily identified in CT/MRI and ultrasound data, in particular in power Doppler ultrasound. Two feature-based rigid approaches are reported in [77] and [78].

For nonrigid intraoperative US registration, we developed and investigated a fast feature-based approach using extracted vessel center lines of the liver. With the use of nonrigid transformations instead of rigid transformations, the accuracy at the vessels was improved by a 5.6, 3.4, and 5.7 mm root mean square difference on three patients. This difference is illustrated in Fig. 2.11. A remaining maximal nonrigid registration error of 6–9 mm at the vessels, 12–15 mm

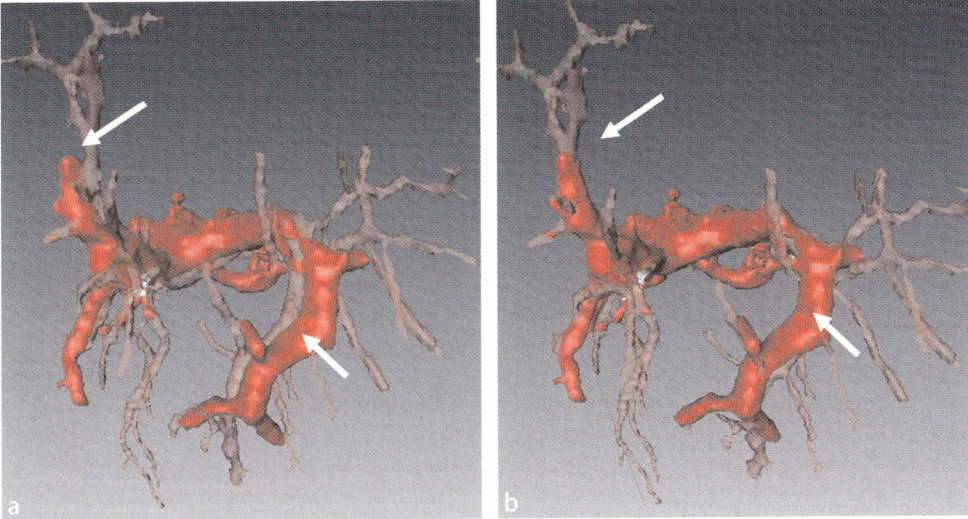

Fig. 2.11a,b Registration of preoperative CT and intraoperative 3D ultrasound data. Portal veins extracted from CT data (*transparent*) and ultrasound data (*opaque*) are shown after rigid (**a**) and nonrigid (**b**) registration

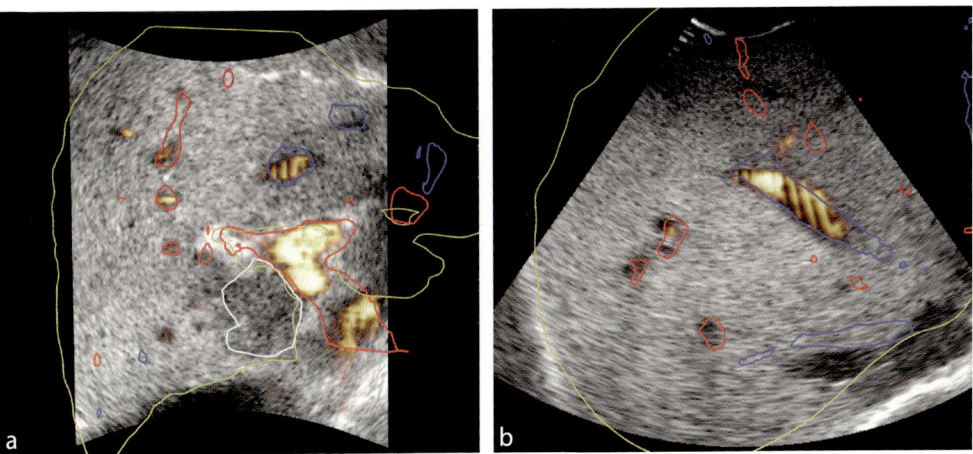

Fig. 2.12a,b Intersection lines of portal veins (*red*), hepatic veins (*blue*), tumor (*white*), and liver surface extracted from preoperative CT data are overlaid on intraoperative ultrasound data

at the tumors, and 16–20 mm at the anterior liver surface was observed (see Fig. 2.12). Until now, the registration was only based on portal veins. For a more detailed description of the algorithm and the achieved results see [79, 80].

The needed extraction of the vessels from the intraoperative US data is the main disadvantage of the method, because to date this cannot be done robustly and fast with an automatic procedure. Hybrid approaches, which fit preoperatively extracted features directly to the intensities of intraoperative image data, might solve this problem. The lack of a time constraint in the preoperative phase allows for precise feature extraction, yielding fast intraoperative registration. Aylward et al. [81] use vessel models and a special distance metric for rigid hybrid registration. We are currently working on nonrigid hybrid approaches.

2.6 Adaptation to Laparoscopic Liver Surgery

To date no clinically applicable navigation system exists for laparoscopic liver surgery. The challenge of organ deformation is similar to open liver surgery, but additional constraints are present because of the minimally invasive access. Transferring conventional navigation approaches to laparoscopic or interventional abdominal procedures is currently being attempted. The main problem in this case is the patient-to-image registration. Obviously, no stereotactic frame or head-set-like construction is suitable for abdominal surgery. Also, external artificial or anatomical landmarks are inappropriate due to the strong deformability of the liver tissue and the insufflation of the abdomen in laparoscopy. In the retroperitoneum, these effects seems to be minor, as shown by Mårvik et al. [41], but even in such applications the accuracy is restricted.

Clearly geometric information from inside the body is needed. In navigated bronchoscopy, endobronchial landmarks such as the main carina are successfully used for registration [82, 83]. These landmarks are identified with an electromagnetically tracked bronchoscope. The accuracy is approximately 5–10 mm. However, internal anatomical landmarks on the liver surface are difficult to define. In addition, they are probably not sufficient for identifying deformations.

Surface scanning provides significantly more geometric information than single points, but for laparoscopy customized small surface scanners are needed. Hayashibe et al. [84] propose a laser-scan laparoscope. A laparoscopic laser device projects laser line beams on the liver surface. These lines are captured by the laparoscopic camera. As the relative positions of the laser device and camera are measured by a tracking system, the 3D position of the laser line can be determined by triangulation.

Such surface scans may support the navigation but probably do not suffice, because the geometry of the anterior part of the liver is not as characteristic as, for example, the brain surface with its sulci. Another question arising is whether scanning at the liver surface is adequate to determine deformations in the depth of the liver. The only way to obtain reliable information from the depth is by intraoperative imaging. Intraoperative ultrasound is already used in laparoscopy and seems to be the most easily integrated into navigated laparoscopic procedures.

The first systems for navigated 2D ultrasound are under investigation in neurosurgery [64, 65] and also for transcutaneous and open liver punctures [66]. The general feasibility for open liver surgery [85] and an adaptation to laparoscopic liver surgery [86] is described, but no accuracy is quantified. Ellsmere et al. [87] propose tracked 2D laparoscopic ultrasound combined with landmark-based registration of CT images. They show that the additional CT images improve the orientation skills of the surgeons on animal tails.

Navigated 3D ultrasound for liver applications has only been reported for an experimental setup of transcutaneous liver ablation [88]. In this study, the advantage of navigated 3D ultrasound over navigated 2D ultrasound is shown. No navigation system based on laparoscopic 3D ultrasound has been developed and investigated so far. The SonoWand as well as our system are principally adaptable to laparoscopic procedures. The crucial point is the availability of laparoscopic 3D ultrasound.

Today no commercial 3D ultrasound device specially dedicated for laparoscopic procedures is available. All four above-mentioned percutaneous 3D ultrasound technologies are principally transferable to laparoscopic applications. But until now only one laparoscopic freehand 3D ultrasound device has been developed [89]. The ultrasound probes currently available for laparoscopy are mostly flexible at the tip. Hence it is not possible to mount a position sensor onto the shaft of the probe outside the body, meaning that optical tracking system cannot be applied, but electromagnetic systems principally can [89]. An alternative is customized small motor-driven or 2D array 3D probes. We conducted preliminary experiments with the 3D endorectal probe of the Voluson 730 machine. The transducer is generally feasible for laparoscopic liver resections. The calibration was carried out on a custom-made US phantom containing three sphere structures.

In addition to the need for laparoscopic 3D ultrasound, appropriate tracking systems are also important for navigated laparoscopy. Position sensors of optical tracking systems can only be measured outside the body, because of the free-line-of-sight condition. For laparoscopy, this means only rigid instruments and rigid 3D ultrasound transducers can be tracked optically. In conventional navigation, electromagnetic tracking systems have played only a minor role until now, because of their smaller measurement volume, lower accuracy, and in particular the interference by metallic objects and magnetic fields in their environment. But recent advances in the interference and the development of very small sensors are promising for use in laparoscopic and endoscopic applications [27]. Successful application in bronchoscopy has been referenced above. But for specific instruments in laparoscopy and in a real OR environment, further investigations are needed.

All conventional and in particular the visualization techniques described for 3D ultrasound navigation can be adapted to laparoscopic navigation. An augmented reality approach would be natural, because a video image of the laparoscopic camera is always available. In a video see-through technique, structures lying beneath the surface of the liver can be visualized.

As in open liver procedures, the problems of transferring preoperative models and plans as well as intraoperatively induced deformations, be they respiration, heart movement, surgery-induced swelling, or cutting, exist in laparoscopy as well. Promising methods have been developed for neurosurgery to compensate brain shift. Unlike the neurosurgical environment where the cranium confines the brain at the initial stage of the surgery, a significant amount of tissue deformation during liver surgery occurs. Because the mobilization of the liver in laparoscopy is not as extensive as in open surgery, the deformations can perhaps be better controlled. Compared to neurosurgery, an accuracy of 5 mm might be sufficient.

Cash et al. [58] attempted to transfer model-updated image-guided surgery methods for brain shift compensation to liver deformations. Their approach consists of a linear elastic model of the liver tissue and liver surface scans as boundary conditions. They report correct localization of subsurface targets within 4 mm in phantom experiments. The main difficulty is to determine the boundary conditions reliably and accurately for the biomechanical model of the liver. The biomechanical model only describes the behavior of the tissue to external forces or restrictions. The actual shape of the liver model is determined by these external conditions such as fixation by ligaments and restriction by other organs or tissues that can freely move. It might also be necessary to measure movements of points inside the liver to better quantify liver deformations. Miniaturized electromagnetic position sensors fitting into catheters or needles are a possibility to measure these point movements.

Navigation systems for laparoscopic liver resections based on 3D ultrasound alone will be available in the near future. They will significantly improve the limitations of laparoscopic procedures such as absence of direct organ palpation by image information from beneath the liver surface and will allow precise resection of tumors. Their clinical value will have to be evaluated. In the medium term, the major challenge, as for all soft tissue navigation approaches, will be to solve the organ deformation issue. On the one hand, fast, robust, and reliable nonrigid registration algorithms are needed, which enable the transfer of preoperative models and resection plans to intraoperative ultrasound data. On the other hand, deformations during the actual resection must be compensated. The combination of intraoperative point, surface, or image measurements with precise biomechanical and possible physiological soft tissue modeling is a promising research direction.

References

1. Marescaux J, Clement JM, Tassetti V, Koehl C, Cotin S, Russier Y, Mutter D, Delingette H, Ayache N (1998) Virtual reality applied to hepatic surgery simulation: the next revolution. Ann Surg 228:627–634
2. Fong Y, Fortner J, Sun RL, Brennan MF, Blumgart LH (1999) Clinical score for predicting recurrence after hepatic resection for metastatic colorectal cancer: analysis of 1001 consecutive cases. Ann Surg 230:309–318
3. Cady B, Jenkins RL, Steele GD Jr, Lewis WD, Stone MD, McDermott WV, Jessup JM, Bothe A, Lalor P, Lovett EJ, Lavin P, Linehan DC (1998) Surgical margin in hepatic resection for colorectal metastasis: a critical and improvable determinant of outcome. Ann Surg 227:566–571
4. Pawlik TM, Scoggins CR, Zorzi D, Abdalla EK, Andres A, Eng C, Curley SA, Loyer EM, Muratore A, Mentha G, Capussotti L, Vauthey JN (2005) Effect of surgical margin status on survival and site of recurrence after hepatic resection for colorectal metastases. Ann Surg 241:715–722
5. Wray CJ, Lowy AM, Mathews JB, Park S, Choe KA, Hanto DW, James LE, Soldano DA, Ahmad SA (2005) The significance and clinical factors associated with a subcentimeter resection of colorectal liver metastases. Ann Surg Oncol 12:374–380
6. Fasel JH, Selle D, Evertsz CJ, Terrier F, Peitgen HO, Gailloud P (1998) Segmental anatomy of the liver: poor correlation with CT. Radiology 206:151–156
7. Lorensen WE, Cline HE (1987) Marching cubes: a high resolution 3D surface construction algorithm. SIGGRAPH 21:163–169
8. Hahn H, Preim B, Selle D, Peitgen HO (2001) Visualization and interaction techniques for the exploration of vascular structures. In: IEEE visualization. IEEE Computer Society, pp 395–402
9. Oeltze S, Preim B (2005) Visualization of vascular structures: method, validation and evaluation. IEEE Trans Med Imag 24:540–548
10. Soler L, Delingette H, Malandain G, Montagnat J, Ayache N, Koehl C, Dourthe O, Malassagne B, Smith M, Mutter D, Marescaux J (2001) Fully automatic anatomical, pathological and functional segmentation from CT scans for hepatic surgery. Comput Aided Surg 21:1344–1357
11. Schenk A, Prause G, Peitgen HO (2000) Efficient semiautomatic segmentation of 3D objects. In: Delp SL, DiGioia AM, Jaramaz B (eds) Medical image computing and computer-assisted intervention (MICCAI), lecture notes in computer science, Vol. 1935, Springer, Berlin New York Heidelberg, pp 186–195
12. Mortensen EN, Barrett WA (1998) Interactive segmentation with intelligent scissors. Graphical Models and Image Processing 60:349–384
13. Turk G, OBrian JF (1999) Shape transformation using variational implicit functions. SIGGRAPH 99:335–342
14. Cootes T, Hill A, Taylor CJ, Haslam J (1994) Use of active shape models for locating structures in medical images. Image Vision Comput 12:355–366
15. Lamecker H, Lange T, Seebass M (2002) A statistical shape model for the liver. In: Dohi T, Kikinis R (eds) Medical image computing and computer-assisted intervention, Vol. 2489, Lecture Notes in Computer Science, Springer, Berlin New York Heidelberg, pp 422–427
16. Lamecker H, Lange T, Seebass M, Eulenstein S, Westerhoff M, Hege HC (2003) Automatic segmentation of the liver for the preoperative planning of resections. In: Westwood JD et al. (eds) Medicine meets virtual reality, Vol. 94. Studies in health technologies and informatics. IOS Press, Amsterdam, pp 171–174
17. Lamecker H, Lange T, Seebass M (2004) Segmentation of the liver using a 3D statistical shape model. Zuse Institute, Berlin. ZIB Technical Report 04–09
18. Lange T, Wenckebach T, Lamecker H, Seebass M, Hünerbein M, Eulenstein S, Gebauer B, Schlag PM (2005) Registration of different phases of contrast-enhanced CT/MRI data for computer-assisted liver surgery planning: evaluation of state-of-the-art methods. Int J Med Robotics Comput Assist Surg 1:6–20
19. Selle D, Preim B, Schenk A, Peitgen HO (2002) Analysis of vasculature for liver surgical planning. IEEE Trans Med Imaging 21:1344–1357

20. Meinzer HP, Thorn M, Cardenas C (2002) Computerized planning of liver surgery – an overview. Comput Graphics 26:569–576
21. Frericks BB, Caldarone FC, Nashan B, Savellano DH, Stamm G, Kirchhoff TD, Shin HO, Schenk A, Selle D, Spindler W, Klempnauer J, Peitgen HO, Galanski M (2004) 3D CT modeling of hepatic vessel architecture and volume calculation in living donated liver transplantation. Eur Radiol 14:326–333
22. Harms J, Bartels M, Bourquain H, Peitgen HO, Schulz T, Kahn T, Hauss J, Fangmann J (2005) Computerized CT-based 3D visualization technique in living related liver transplantation. Transplant Proc 37:1059–1062
23. Hogemann D, Stamm G, Shin H, Oldhafer KJ, Schlitt HJ, Selle D, Peitgen HO (2000) Individual planning of liver surgery interventions with a virtual model of the liver and its associated structures. Radiologe 40:267–273
24. Oldhafer KJ, Hogemann D, Stamm G, Raab R, Peitgen HO, Galanski M (1999) 3-dimensional (3-D) visualization of the liver for planning extensive liver resections. Chirurg 70:233–238
25. Preim B, Bourquian H, Selle D, Peitgen HO, Oldhafer KJ (2002) Resection proposals for oncologic liver surgery based on vascular territories. In: Lemke HU, Vannier, MW, Inamura K, Farman AG (eds) Computer assisted radiology and surgery (CARS). Springer, Berlin New York Heidelberg, pp 353–358
26. Lang H, Radtke A, Hindenach M, Schroeder T, Frühauf NR, Malgó M, Bourquain H, Peitgen HO, Oldhafer KJ, Broelsch CE (2005) Impact of virtual tumor resection and computer-assisted risk analysis on operation planning and intraoperative strategy in major hepatic resection. Arch Surg 140:629–638
27. Schicho K, Figl M, Donat M, Birkfellner W, Seemann R, Wagner A, Bergmann H, Ewers R (2005) Stability of miniature electromagnetic tracking systems. Phys Med Biol 50:2089–2098
28. Peters TM (2000) Image guided surgery: from X-rays to virtual reality. Comput Methods Biomech Biomed Eng 4:27–57
29. Knott PD, Maurer CR, Gallivan R, Roh HJ, Citardi MJ (2004) The impact of fiducial distribution on headset-based registration in image-guided sinus surgery. Otolaryngol Head Neck Surg 131:666–672
30. Maurer CR, Fitzpatrick JM, Wang MY, Galloway RL, Maciunas RJ (1997) Registration of head volume images using implantable fiducial markers. IEEE Trans Med Imaging 16:447–462
31. Besl PJ, McKay ND (1992) A method for registration of 3-D shapes. IEEE PAMI 14:239–256
32. Raabe A, Krishan R, Wolff R, Hermann E, Zimmermann M, Seifert V (2002) Laser surface scanning for patient registration in intracranial image-guided surgery. Neurosurgery 50:797–803
33. Marmulla R, Lüth T, Mühling J, Hassfeld S (2004) Automated laser registration in image-guided surgery: evaluation of the correlation between laser scan resolution and navigation accuracy. Int J Oral Maxillofac Surg 33:642–648
34. Azuma RT (1997) A survey of augmented reality. Presence: Teleoperators and Virtual Environments 6:355–385
35. Wirtz CR, Knauth M, Hassfeld S, Tronnier VM, Albert FK, Bonsanto M, Kunze S (1998) Neuronavigation – first experiences with three different commercially available systems. Zentralbl Neurochir 59:14–22
36. State A, Linvingston MA, Hirota G, Garret WF, Whitton MC, Fuchs H (1996) Technologies for augmented-reality systems: realizing ultrasound-guided needle biopsies. In: SIGGRAPH 96 Conference Proceedings, ACM SIGGRAPH, Addison Wesley, pp 439–446
37. Grimson WEL, Lozano-Perez T, Wells WM, Ettinger GJ, White SJ, Kikinis R (1996) An automatic registration method for frameless stereotaxy, image guided surgery, and enhanced reality visualization. IEEE Trans Med Imaging 15:129–140
38. Fichtinger G, Deguet A, Masamune K, Fischer G, Balogh E, Mathieu H, Taylor RH, Fayad LM, Zinreich SJ (2004) Needle Insertion in CT scanner with image overlay–cadaver studies. In: Medical image computing and computer assisted intervention (MICCAI). Vol. 3217, Lecture Notes in Computer Science (LNCS), Springer, Berlin New York, Heidelberg, pp 795–803
39. Schwald B, Seibert H, Schnaider M, Wesarg S, Röddiger S, Dogan S (2004) Implementation and evaluation of an augmented reality system supporting minimal invasive interventions. In: Vol. Workshop AMI-ARCS 2004, pp 41–48

40. Hoppe H, Eggers G, Heurich T, Raczkowsky J, Marmulla R, Wörn H, Hassfeld S, Moctezuma JL (2003) Projector based visualization for intraoperative navigation: first clinical results. In: Lemke HU, Vannier, MW, Inamura K, Farman AG, Doi K, Reiber JHC (eds) Proc Comput Assist Radiol Surg (CARS) pp 771
41. Mårvik R, Langø T, Tangen GA, Andersen JO, Kaspersen JH, Ystgaard B, Sjølie E, Fougner R, Fjøsne HE, Nagelhus Hernes TA (2004) Laparoscopic navigation pointer for three-dimensional image-guided surgery. Surg Endosc 18:1242–1248
42. Kaspersen JH, Sjølie E, Wesche J, Asland J, Lundbom J, Odegård A, Lindseth F, Nagelhus Hernes TA (2003) 3D ultrasound based navigation combined with preoperative CT during abdominal interventions: A feasibility study. Cardiovasc Interv Radiol 26:347–356
43. Banovac F, Tang J, Xu S, Lindisch D, Chung HY, Levy EB, Chang T, McCullough MF, Yaniv Z, Wood BJ, Cleary K (2005) Precision targeting of liver lesions using a novel electromagnetic navigation device in physiologic phantom and swine. Med Phys 32:2698–2705
44. Wallace MJ, Gupta S, Hicks ME (2006) Out-of-plane computed-tomography-guided biopsy using a magnetic-field-based navigation system. Cardiovasc Interv Radiol 29:108–113
45. Nicolau SA, Garcia A, Pennec X, Soler L, Ayache N (2005) An augmented reality system to guide radio-frequency tumour ablation. Comput Animat Virtual World 16:1–10
46. Nicolau SA, Pennec X, Soler L, Ayache N (2005) A complete augmented reality guidance system for liver punctures: first clinical evaluation. In: Duncan J, Gerig G (eds) Medical image computing and computer-assisted intervention (MICCAI). Vol 3749, Lecture Notes in Computer Science, Springer, Berlin New York, Heidelberg, pp 539–547
47. Herline AJ, Herring JL, Stefansic JD, Chapman WC, Galloway RL, Dawant BM (2000) Surface registration for use in interactive, image-guided liver surgery. Comput Aided Surg 5:11–17
48. Cash DM, Sinha TK, Chapman WC, Terawaki H, Dawant BM, Galloway RL, Miga MI (2003) Incorporation of a laser range scanner into image-guided liver surgery: surface acquisition, registration, and tracking. Med Phys 30:1671–1682
49. Sinha TK, Dawant BM, Duay V, Cash DM, Weil RJ, Thompson RC, Weaver KD, Miga M (2005) A method to track cortical surface deformations using a laser range scanner. IEEE Trans Med Imaging 24:767–781
50. Sun H, Roberts DW, Farid H, Wu Z, Hartov A, Paulsen KD (2005) Cortical surface tracking using a stereoscopic operating microscope. Neurosurgery 56:86–95
51. Miga M, Roberts DW, Kennedy FE, Platinek LA, Hartov A, Lunn KE, Paulsen KD (2001) Modelling of retraction and resection for intraoperative updating of images. Neurosurgery 49:75–85
52. Picinbono G, Delingette H, Ayache N (2003) Nonlinear anisotropic elasticity for real-time surgery simulation. Graphical Models 65:305–321
53. Paulsen KD, Miga MI, Kennedy FE, Hoopes PJ, Hartov A, Roberts DW (1999) A computational model for tracking subsurface tissue deformation during stereotactic neurosurgery. IEEE Trans Biomed Eng 46:213–225
54. Miller K (2000) Constitutive modelling of abdominal organs. J Biomech 33:367–373
55. Miller K, Chinzei K, Orssengo G, Bednarz P (2000) Mechanical properties of brain tissue in-vivo: experiment and computer simulation. J Biomech 33:1369–1376
56. Sun H, Lunn KE, Farid H, Wu Z, Roberts DW, Hartov A, Paulsen KD (2005) Stereopsis-guided brain shift compensation. IEEE Trans Med Imaging 24:1039–1052
57. Miga MI, Cash DM, Cao Z, Galloway RL, Dawant BM, Chapman WC (2003) Intraoperative registration of the liver for image-guided surgery using laser range scanning and deformable models. In: Medical Imaging 2003: visualization, image-guided procedures and display. Vol. 5029, Proceedings of the SPIE, pp 350–359
58. Cash DM, Miga MI, Sinha TK, Galloway RL, Chapman WC (2005) Compensating for intraoperative soft-tissue deformations using incomplete surface data and finite elements. IEEE Trans Med Imaging 24:1479–1491
59. Lunn KE, Paulsen KD, Roberts DW, Kennedy FE, Hartov A, West J (2003) Displacement estimation with co-registered ultrasound for image guided neurosurgery: a quantitative in vivo porcine study. IEEE Trans Med Imaging 22:1358–1368
60. Nimsky C, Ganslandt O, Hastreiter P (2001) Intraoperative compensation for brain shift. Surg Neurol 43:357–364

61. Nabavi A, Black PM, Gering DT, Westin CF, Mehta V, Perolizzi RS, Ferrant M, Warfield SK, Hata N, Schwartz RB, Wells WM, Kikinis R, Jolesy FA (2001) Serial intraoperative MR imaging of brain shift. Neurosurgery 48:787–798
62. Gebhard F, Weidner A, Liener UC, Stockle U, Arand M (2004) Navigation at the spine. Injury 35 [Suppl 1]:S-A:35–34
63. Nolte LP, Beutler T (2004) Basic principles of CAOS. Injury 35:S-A6–S-A16
64. Trobaugh JW, Richard WD, Smith KR, Bucholz RD (1994) Frameless stereotactic ultrasonography: method and applications. Comput Med Imaging Graph 18:235–246
65. Comeau RM, Sadikot AF, Fenster A, Peters TM (2000) Intraoperative ultrasound for guidance and tissue shift correction in image-guided neurosurgery. Med Phys 27:787–800
66. Birth M, Iblher P, Hildebrand P, Nolde J, Bruch HP (2003) Ultrasound-guided interventions using magnetic field navigation. First experiences with Ultra-Guide 2000 under operative conditions. Ultraschall Med 24:90–95
67. Tuthill TA, Krücker JF, Fowlkes JB, Carson PL (1998) Automated three-dimensional US frame positioning computed from elevational speckle decorrelation. Radiology 209:575–282
68. Prager RW, Gee Ah, Treece GM, Berman L (2003) Sensorless freehand 3D ultrasound using regression of the echo intensity. Ultrasound Med Biol 29.437 446
69. Mercier L, Lango T, Lindseth F, Collins L (2005) A review of calibration techniques for freehand 3-D ultrasound systems. Ultrasound Med Biol 31:449–471
70. Gronningsaeter A, Kleven A, Ommedal S, Aarseth TE, Lie T, Lindseth F, Lango T, Unsgard G (2000) SonoWand, an ultrasound-based neuronavigation system. Neurosurgery 47:1373–1379
71. Unsgaard G, Ommedal S, Muller T, Gronningsaeter A, Nagelhus Hernes TA (2002) Neuronavigation by intraoperative three-dimensional ultrasound: initial experience during brain tumor resection. Neurosurgery 50:804–812
72. Lindseth F, Langø T, Bang J, Hernes T (2002) Accuracy evaluation of a 3D ultrasound-based neuronavigation system. Comput Aided Surg 7:197–222
73. Roche A, Pennec X, Malandain G, Ayache N (2001) Rigid registration of 3-D ultrasound With MR images: a new approach combining intensity and gradient information. IEEE Trans Med Imaging 20:1038–1049
74. Slomka PJ, Mandel J, Downey D, Fenster A (2001) Evaluation of voxel-based registration of 3-D power Doppler ultrasound and 3-D magnetic resonance angiographic images of carotid arteries. Ultrasound Med Biol 27:945–955
75. Pennec X, Cachier P, Ayache N (2003) Tracking brain deformations in time sequences of 3D US images. Pattern Recognition Lett 24:801–813
76. Letteboer M, Willems P, Viergever MA, Niessen WJ (2003) Non-rigid registration of 3D ultrasound images of brain tumours acquired during neurosurgery. In: Ellis RE, Peters TM (eds) Medical image computing and computer-assisted intervention. Vol. 2879, Springer, Berlin New York Heidelberg, pp 408–415
77. Porter BC, Rubens DJ, Strang JG, Smith J, Totterman S, Parker KJ (2001) Three-dimensional registration and fusion of ultrasound and MRI using major vessels as fiducial markers. IEEE Trans Med Imaging 20:354–359
78. Penney GP, Blackall JM, Hamady MS, Sabharwal T, Adam A, Hawkes DJ (2004) Registration of freehand 3D ultrasound and magnetic resonance liver images. Med Image Anal 8:81–91
79. Lange T, Eulenstein S, Hünerbein M, Schlag PM (2003) Vessel-based non-rigid registration of MR/CT and 3D ultrasound for navigation in liver surgery. Comput Aided Surg 8:228–240
80. Lange T, Eulenstein S, Hünerbein M, Lamecker H, Schlag PM (2004) Augmenting intraoperative 3D ultrasound with preoperative models for navigation in liver surgery. In: Barillot C, Haynor DR, Hellier P (eds) Medical image computing and computer-assisted intervention. Vol. 3217, Lecture Notes in Computer Science, Springer, Berlin New York Heidelberg, pp 534–541
81. Aylward SR, Jomier J, Weeks S, Bullitt E (2003) Registration and analysis of vascular images. Int J Comput Vision 55:123–138
82. Schwarz Y, Mehta AC, Ernst A, Herth F, Engel A, Besser D, Becker HD (2003) Electromagnetic navigation during flexible bronchoscopy. Respiration 70:516–522

83. Hautmann H, Schneider A, Pinkau T, Peltz F, Feussner H (2005) Electromagnetic catheter navigation during bronchoscopy: validation of a novel method by conventional fluoroscopy. Chest 128:382–387
84. Hayashibe M, Suzuki N, Hattori A, Nakamura Y (2002) Intraoperative fast 3D shape recovery of abdominal organs in laparoscopy. In: Dohi T, Kikinis R (eds). Medical image computing and computer-assisted intervention. Vol. 2489, Lecture Notes in Computer Science (LNCS), Springer, Berlin New York Heidelberg, pp 356–363
85. Birth M, Kleemann M, Hildebrand P, Bruch HP (2004) Intraoperative online navigation of dissection of the hepatical tissue – a new dimension in liver surgery. In: Lemke HU, Vannier MW, Inamura K, Farman AG, Doi K, Reiber JHC (eds) Computer assisted radiology and surgery (CARS). Vol. 1268, ICS, Elsevier, Amsterdam, pp 770–774
86. Kleemann M, Hildebrand P, Keller R, Bruch HP, Birth M (2004) Laparoscopic ultrasound navigation in liver surgery – technical aspects and feasibility. In: Lemke HU, Vannier MW, Inamura K, Farman AG, Doi K, Reiber JHC (eds) Computer assisted radiology and surgery (CARS). Vol. 1268, ICS, Elsevier, Amsterdam, pp 793–796
87. Ellsmere J, Stoll J, Rattner D, Brooks D, Kane R, Wells WM, Kikinis R, Vosburgh K (2003) A navigation system for augmenting laparoscopic ultrasound. In: Ellis RE, Peters TM (eds). Medical image computing and computer assisted intervention. Vol. 2879, Springer, Berlin New York Heidelberg, pp 184–191
88. Sjølie E, Kaspersen JH, Wesche J, Lindseth F, Hernes T (2001) Minimal invasive abdominal surgery based on ultrasound vision, possible? In: Lemke HU, Vannier, MW, Inamura K, Farman AG, Doi K (eds) Computer assisted radiology and surgery. Vol. 1230, Elsevier, Amsterdam, pp 39–44
89. Harms J, Feussner H, Baumgartner M, Schneider A, Donhauser M, Wessels G (2001) Three-dimensional navigated laparoscopic ultrasonography. Surg Endosc 15:1459–1462

Part II Methods of Minimally Invasive Tumor Therapies

3 Radiofrequency Ablation: The Percutaneous Approach

Philippe Pereira, Andreas Boss, Stephen Clasen,
Cecile Gouttefangeas, Diethard Schmidt, Claus D. Claussen

Recent Results in Cancer Research, Vol. 167
© Springer-Verlag Berlin Heidelberg 2006

3.1 Introduction

Percutaneous image-guided tumor ablation using the thermal procedure has increased in importance over the last 10 years into a promising, minimally invasive therapy strategy for the treatment of primary and secondary liver malignancies [1, 2]. This procedure was primarily used in neurosurgery as early as the 1960s in order to destroy locally small areas of the brain [3]. In the 1990s, radiofrequency (RF) ablation of malignant liver tumors was first studied within feasibility studies [4, 5]. Clinical studies with long-term results have been reported beginning with the end of the 1990s [6–9].

In the search for an alternative therapy for nonsurgical patients, a whole range of minimally invasive therapy procedures have been developed in the last few years: RF ablation, interstitial laser thermal therapy (LITT), microwaves (MWs), high-intensity focused ultrasound (HIFU), and cryotherapy. The use of laser therapy in the case of colorectal metastases has shown promising results [10]. The largest experience with MW therapy has been seen in Japan. However, one disadvantage of MW therapy is the geometry of the thermally induced lesion obtained by this procedure: small and ellipsoidal, which often does not correspond to the geometry of liver tumors [11]. HIFU therapy is still in its experimental stages and, at present, only small inadequate coagulations are possible. However, its main advantage will be its noninvasiveness, since high-energy ultrasound waves are applied via an US transmitter without puncture [12]. Finally, cryoablation, which has been used for several years in surgery, has the disadvantage for a percutaneous approach of working with large-diameter applicators, which renders cryotherapy mainly an intraoperative modality. However, it is more complicated and cost-intensive compared to RF ablation [14]. Comparing all the thermal ablation methods currently available, RF ablation is by far the most frequently used worldwide. An explanation for this can be seen in its effectiveness in destroying the tumor tissue as well as the low complication rate. Another reason is also its reduced technical demand in comparison to that of cryoablation or laser technology [15–17].

3.2 Principles of Radiofrequency and Thermal Bioeffects

The first description of a use of local heating for coagulation of tissue can be found in early Egyptian and Greek literature. In 1891, D'Arsonval described the warm induction in biological tissues through RF waves [18]. The principle was based on closed electricity circuit between a RF generator and a patient. The RF waves were emitted from an active noninsulated electrode and then diverted to one or more neutral electrodes. In the 1970s, Organ et al. discovered that by using low electric energy, an intracell ionic movement was induced resulting from the alternating current, with the consequences of inducing a frictional heating of the tissue surrounding the applicator tip [19]. At the beginning of the 1990s, two research groups modified the RF systems to be able to induce large coagulation in liver tissue [5, 20]. The radius of the coagulation was, however, limited to 1 cm. The further development of the RF technique had, nevertheless, shown that together with an increase in applied energy, a prolonged ablation time, and an enlargement of the active electrode tip, the volume of the coagulation necrosis can be increased by up to 400% in the case of liver tissue [21, 22].

For image-guided tumor treatment using RF ablation, a RF applicator is positioned in the tumor by using imaging for guidance [23]. The RF applicator consists of a metal shaft, which is electrically insulated, and a noninsulated so-called active electrode tip. The RF generator delivers a sinus-form high-frequency alternating current (375–480 kHz) which, via the active electrode, is emitted into the surrounding tissue. A RF field of tension between the electrode tip and the neutral electrode – placed on patient's skin – is therefore built up so that the current can run freely backward and forward. In comparison to the large area of the neutral electrode, the active part of the RF electrode only shows a small area in the field. Through this, the tension and the current thickness in the immediate region surrounding the electrode tip are high, leading to warmth through friction via the intracellular ionic movements. Coagulation necrosis takes place in the surrounding tissue with a temperature higher than 60 °C [24]. The numerous parameters that play a part in the volume of coagulation were previously reported by Pennes using a complicated formula [25]. This equation – also known as bio-heat transfer equation – can be represented using the following simplified approach:

Extent of coagulation necrosis = applied energy × local tissue interactions – heat loss

An increase in temperature from 40 °C to 42–45 °C renders the cells more susceptible to damage [26, 27]. When cells are exposed to temperatures of over 45 °C, irreversible damage takes place after 1 h [28]. A further increase in temperature to 50–52 °C reduces this time to 2 min, in which a cytotoxic effect leads to irreversible cell death.

With temperatures between 60 °C and 100 °C, an immediate irreversible protein denaturation with release of mitochondrial key enzymes occurs, as well as a destruction of the DNA structure [21, 24, 29]. These high temperatures result in coagulation necrosis. The histopathological criteria for a coagulation necrosis may not, however, have been met immediately after ablation, since thermally induced coagulation is an active process taking several days up to 2–3 weeks. Therefore, the strength of statement of a tissue biopsy after ablation in order to confirm a successful tumor ablation is limited if performed immediately after thermoablation. Temperatures over 105 °C cause a build up of gas and carbonization in the exposed tissue. Therefore, temperatures between 65 °C and 100 °C are considered optimal.

The friction-induced heat alters tissue resistance through the production of coagulative necrosis. If temperatures of 90 °C or more are too quickly achieved, then carbonization and vaporization processes occur, resulting in a noticeable increase in the electrical resistance in the tissue. The electrical conductivity and, therefore, also the heat conduction are, however, independent from the resistance of the tissue. Therefore, the size of the coagulation is automatically limited. The increase in resistance in the tissue must be avoided in the case of RF ablation because the thermally produced lesion will remain small. It was written in the 1990s that by using single electrodes for RF therapy, a maximum coagulation diameter of 1.6 cm is possible. Subsequently, the clinical use of this method did initially have its limitations for liver tumor therapy [22]. The technical developments of the RF devices have shown, however, that a therapeutically relevant coagulation diameter can nowadays be achieved in a reproducible manner [30]. In accordance to the bio-heat equation, this strategy is based on the one hand on the increase in energy deposition in the tissue, and on the other hand, on the method of the energy transmission. Also, to be accounted for is an improvement in the heat conduction into the tissue and, finally, the reduction in the tumor tolerance to heat. An additional option is the prevention of too much heat loss through variation of the blood circulation.

3.3 Radiofrequency Systems

3.3.1 Radiofrequency Generators

Several RF generators are approved bt the FDA or CE for clinical use. These commercially available systems are divided into monopolar, bipolar, and multipolar RF devices (Table 3.1).

The monopolar RF generators use a power output of either 60W (HiTT Elekrotom 106, Berchtold-Integra ME, Plainsboro, NJ, USA), or 200 W (RF 3000, Boston Scientific, Mountain View, CA, USA, and Cool Tip, Valley Lab, Boulder, CO, USA), and at least 250 W (Model 1500x, RITA Medical Systems, Mountain View, CA, USA). The control of an ablation course, and with it the amount of energy deposition, is based on resistance (Berchtold, Boston Scientific, Valley Lab.) or temperature (RITA). It must be noted that a standard protocol for each of the RF systems exists for ablation in the liver. However, clinical experience has shown that the standard protocol must be adapted to each individual tumor. Therefore, the responsibility for a successful tumor ablation lies in the hands of the interventional physician, who ultimately has to set the parameters for ablation length, ablation probe, and power output and the number of applicator repositionings that may be necessary to treat a tumor with a safety margin.

3.3.2 Monopolar Ablation Devices

Initially, RF ablation in neurosurgery and cardiology was mainly performed with monopolar needle-like electrodes. Using these applicators, Goldberg et al. achieved a coagulation diameter of up to 1.6 cm [22]. The correlation between the size of coagulation and the electrode length, temperature, and ablation length parameters were tested in experimental ex-vivo liver and muscle tissues [22, 31]. For longer ablation times, an increase in a coagulation diameter of 3.0–4.0 cm was observed. The length of the active electrode had a linear effect on the length diameter of the coagulation but not always on the width diam-

Table 3.1 Technical data of commercially available radiofrequency generators

RF-System	HiTT 106 Berchtold-Integra	Cool Tip ValleyLab	RF 3000 Boston Scientific	Model 1500x RITA	Celon Power-Olympus
Strength	60 W	200 W	200 W	250 W	250 W
Frequency	375 kHz	480 kHz	480 kHz	460 kHz	470 kHz
Monitoring of ablation	Tissue resistance	Tissue resistance	Tissue resistance	Tissue resistance and temperature	Tissue resistance
Energy application	Monopolar	Monopolar	Monopolar	Monopolar	Bipolar or multipolar
Applicator: diameter	1.7 mm	1.6 mm / 3×1.6 mm	2.5 mm	2.2 mm	1.8 mm
Applicator: Configuration and active part	Straight 1.5 cm	Straight Single/cluster 3 cm/2.5 cm	Umbrella 4 cm	Christmas-tree 5 cm/7 cm	Straight 4 cm
Applicator:	Perfused	Internally cooled (single/cluster)	Expandable	Expandable	Internally cooled
Type and MR compatibility	Yes	Yes (single and cluster)	Yes (3.5 cm)	Yes (Xl)	Yes (bipolar and multipolar)

eter [32]. Therefore, the optimal length of the active electrode was considered to be 3 cm. The increase in the electrode diameter from 24G to 12G increased the coagulation diameter from 0.7 cm to 1.8 cm.

3.3.3 Cooled and Perfused Monopolar Needle-Like Applicators

3.3.3.1 Internally Cooled Single Applicator (Valley Lab)

The ablation probe is internally cooled via two lumina that are perfused with water during energy application (Fig. 3.1a). The cooling of the applicator delays a premature carbonization along the needle shaft by removing the heat and therefore allows for the deposit of more energy compared with conventional noncooled electrodes [31, 35, 36]. Goldberg et al. used an 18G electrode with maximal cooling in the region of the active electrode of $15 \pm 2\,°C$. Under these conditions, an energy flow from 350, 550, 750, and 1 100 mA with different active applicator lengths could be applied for a total duration of 60 min. Carbonization was not recorded. The short axis of coagulation obtained was 2.5, 3.0, 4.5, and 4.4 cm for active electrode lengths of 1, 2, 3, and 4 cm, respectively. In vivo studies using internally cooled electrodes were conducted on muscle and liver tissue. The short coagulation diameter rose with the increase in deposited energy from 1.8 to 5.4 cm. Following clinical application, Solbiati et al. reported that coagulation transverse diameters of 2.8 ± 0.4 cm with single electrodes were achievable [4].

3.3.3.2 Internally Cooled Cluster Applicator (Valley Lab)

Increased coagulation diameter can also be obtained by using clustered applicators: three individually, internally cooled single electrodes grouped with a distance of 0.5 cm (Fig. 3.1b). In an experimental study, cluster applicators were used with different ablation times ranging from 5 to 60 min in both ex vivo and in vivo experiments [30]. The transverse diameter of coagulation during ex vivo liver ablation of 15, 30, and 45 min were 4.7, 6.2, and 7.0 cm, respectively. For comparison, a coagulation diameter of 2.7 cm ($p < 0.01$) was achieved in 45 min using a single electrode. In in vivo liver and muscle tissue experiments, with an ablation time of 12 min, a coagulation transverse diameter of 3.1 and 7.3 cm, respectively, was obtained. This means a volume increase from 83% to 608% for these in vivo muscle tissues using the cluster applicator in comparison with a single electrode.

3.3.3.3 Perfused Single Applicator (Berchtold-Integra HiTT)

This principle of perfused electrodes is based on a continuous saline perfusion during the RF ablation through two to four micropores located at the tip of the active electrode (Fig. 3.1c). Since resistance is recorded during ablation, an increase in this resistance produces a saline bolus release via the micropores in order to keep the resistance in low values. Approximately 75 ml/h saline solution is perfused into the tissue by 30 W, and 120 ml/h by 60 W. Ex vivo examinations have shown that a coagulation diameter of 6.0 cm is feasible. However, the shape of the thermally induced lesion was irregular and not reproducible [37]. Initial in vivo experiments show that a successful tumor ablation is possible in skilled hands when the tumor and the applicator position are strictly taken into account [38].

3.3.4 Monopolar Expandable Applicators

The coagulation volume of the monopolar electrode could, of course, be increased by altering of the length of the active electrode. However, thermal coagulation produced with single applicators normally has a rather unfortunate cylindrical form that is unlike the usual ball shape of a tumor. Therefore, a strategy was formulated implementing several monopolar electrodes. Goldberg et al. showed in two ex vivo experiments, which, with the use of two to five monopolar applicators, larger areas of necrotic tissue can be produced compared to with a single conventional electrode. A further result of this was the simultaneous energy transmission with greater efficiency cthan switching all electrodes successively [33]. Two expandable RF applicators are commercially available.

3.3.4.1 Expandable LeVeen Applicator (Boston Scientific)

This device involves an expandable umbrella electrode that consists of a hollow needle with a diameter from 14–16G and 10–12 expandable prongs (Fig. 3.1d). When the prongs are fully extended, the diameter reaches 4 cm. In an animal experiment, LeVeen et al. were able to achieve a spherical coagulation with a transverse diameter of up to 3.5 cm using an umbrella electrode initially at 50 W, with an ablation time of 5 min. However, when the power was increased step by step to 80 W, the total ablation time was 12 min [34].

3.3.4.2 Expandable Starburst Applicator (RITA Medical Systems)

The prongs of this applicator are arranged in a hook-like Christmas tree form as opposed to the umbrella like configuration of the LeVeen applicator. The applicator consists of a hollow needle with a 14G diameter and nine expandable prongs (Fig. 3.1e). The diameter of the fully expanded electrode reaches 5 cm (Starburst Xl), although further developments using a larger diameter (7 cm; Starburst XLi) are now available. The energy deposition with this device is controlled by temperature.

3.3.5 Bipolar Radiofrequency Applicators

The single-needle bipolar technique uses a positive (active) and a negative (so-called grounding pad for monopolar systems) electrode that are both integrated into an applicator. This is a different strategy compared to monopolar RF systems, which apply an alternating electric current between a monopolar electrode placed in the target tissue and large dispersive electrodes. In bipolar RF ablation, the electrical circuit is closed between two electrodes placed in proximity and no grounding pads are required. As opposed to the monopolar system, the tissue is heated around the positive as well as the negative electrode. Clinical experience with the bipolar system for tumor therapy is, however, still limited [39]. McGahan et al. examined coagulation that was produced using two monopolar applicators. The short axis of the coagulation was 1.4 cm, and the length diameter 4 cm [40]. Another device for bipolar RF ablation includes both electrodes on the same shaft [41]. A recent commercially available RF device (Celon Lab Power, Olympus-Celon AG, Teltow, Germany), providing a maximum power output of 250 W, enables application of RF energy in bipolar and multipolar modes. RF energy is deposited by using internally cooled applicators. With this device, two electrodes are located on the same shaft of the applicator for bipolar RF ablation (Fig. 3.1f). The electric field is orientated parallel to the bipolar applicator shaft. When more than one bipolar applicator is connected to the RF generator, the electrical current is automatically applied in a multipolar mode. Hence the main electric fields are orientated parallel to the bipolar applicators but cross the tissue between the applicators. The combination of three bipolar applicators is supposed to lead to a more spherical zone of coagulation compared to two bipolar applicators.

3.3.6 Pulsed Radiofrequency Energy Deposition (Valley Lab)

Another strategy in the optimization of RF ablation is obtainable by the pulsed energy modus. The periodical increase and decrease of high energy (up to 2000 mA) leads to a cooling in the immediate region of the active electrode tip without a relevant loss of temperature at the periphery. The combination of an internally cooled cluster applicator with pulsed energy deposition has shown that significantly larger coagulation areas are possible with a diameter of up to 4.5 cm ex

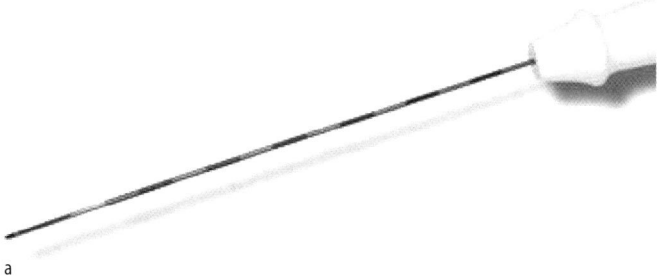

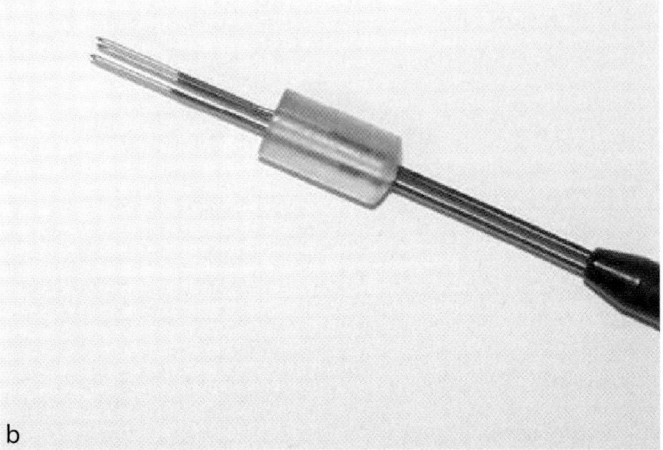

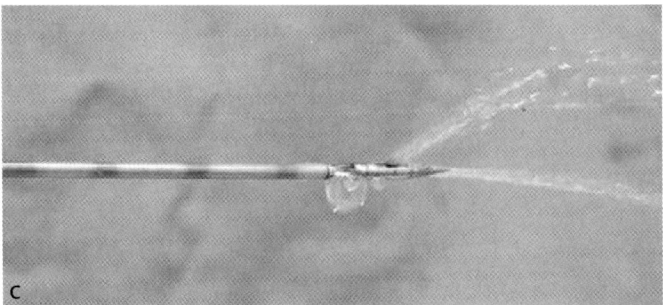

Fig. 3.1 a Internally cooled single applicator with a 3-cm noninsulated "active" tip. b Internally cooled cluster applicator with three single electrodes (active tip, 2.5 cm) grouped together with a distance of 0.5 cm. c The perfusion applicator with a continuous saline perfusion during the RF ablation via the micropores at the tip of the active electrode. d Twelve-tined expandable applicator with an umbrella configuration. e Applicator with nine expandable electrodes that are arranged in a Christmas-tree form as opposed to the umbrella-like electrode arrangement from Boston Scientific. f The needle-like bipolar applicator uses an active and a negative electrode that are both integrated in the same RF needle

3 Radiofrequency Ablation: The Percutaneous Approach

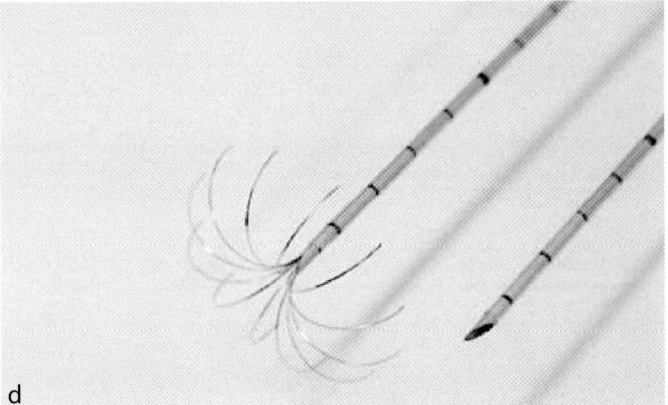

d

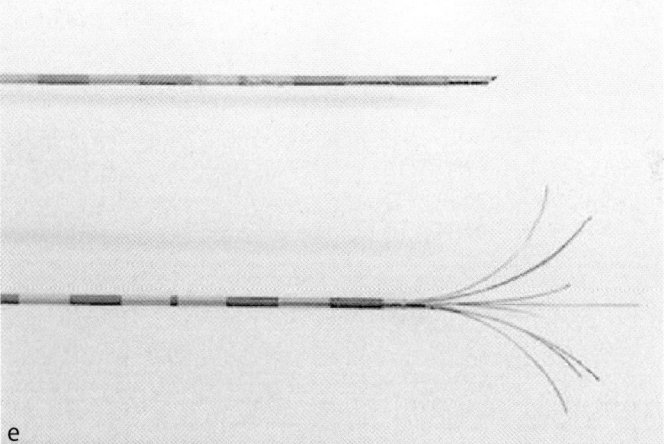

e

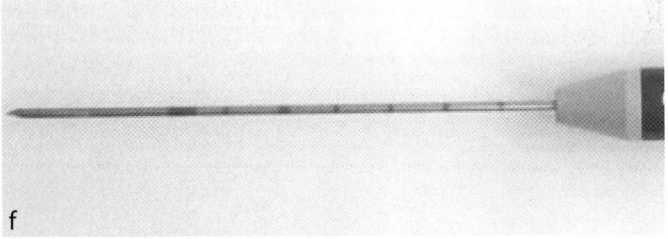

f

vivo [42]. The algorithm for a pulsed RF ablation appears as follows: an increase in the resistance over 20 ohms of the initial value reduces the energy output (by 100 mA). After the decrease in resistance, an automatic new increase of power up to the initial value after maximal 15 s then follows. The use of the cluster electrode in combination with pulsed RF energy transmission shows that in vivo coagulation with short axis diameters of 4.0 cm is achievable at 2000 mA.

3.4 Heat Conduction and Clinical Challenges

3.4.1 Neutral Electrodes and Skin Burns

Due to the trend in using high-power generators (250–400 W) for thermal therapy, serious skin burns in the region of the neutral electrodes can be a danger. Goldberg et al. have systematically varied the number of neutral electrodes (1, 2, or 3), the position of the neutral electrodes (horizontal, vertical, or diagonal), and the distance between the neutral electrodes and the active electrodes (10–50 cm) in in vivo tests. Different neutral electrodes (foil-type or net-type) were implemented [45]. Third-degree burns were reported at temperatures of more than 52 °C. No burns could be detected when the distance between the RF applicator and neutral pads was greater than 25 cm.

3.4.2 Tissue Conductivity

The conclusions of the numerous ex vivo experimental tests cannot be directly adapted for in vivo use [1]. The problem of heat loss through tissue perfusion and/or permanent blood flow in the liver tissue may be an important factor of error in the transposition of ex vivo experience to in vivo circumstances. This difference between ex vivo and in vivo results was previously reported by Penne in his tissue bio-heat equation and must be taken into account for in vivo thermal ablations [25]. A further limitation lies in the different blood supplies of different tumor tissues, which obviously has a significant influence on the heat distribution in the tumor mass. This is the reason why there are attempts to alter the physiological perfusion of the tumor tissue, whereby two basic strategies can be followed: an increased heating of the exposed tissue or an increase in the coagulated volume for a constant energy deposition. An increase in tissue heating can be achieved by a previous injection of saline solution or magnetic particles in order to increase tissue conductivity [43]. An improvement in heat conduction from the active electrode into the periphery is also possible with a continuous saline solution flow [41, 44].

3.4.3 Saline Solution Injection for Optimizing Heat Conduction

The electrical conductivity in tissue governs the energy deposition with the precondition of a constant energy application. Hence, several working groups have already examined the influence of saline solution injection on necrosis volume during RF ablation [37, 44]. Miao et al. achieved a coagulation diameter of 5.5 cm after 12 min of energy deposit with a 5% NaCl solution and a perfusion amount of 1 ml/min. Subsequent tests with different NaCl concentrations followed. In animal tests, Goldberg et al. confirmed that the previous injection of 6 ml of a 38.5% NaCl solution led to a near doubling of the coagulation short-axis diameter from 3.6 cm to 7.0 cm.

3.4.4 Tissue Blood Flow

A challenge for the RF ablation of liver malignancies is the dual blood flow of the liver. Artery and particularly portal vein blood flow leads to a significant loss of produced heat through transport (perfusion-mediated cooling) or direct cooling (the heat sink effect), so-called thermal convection. This heat loss markedly reduces in vivo the size of the coagulative necrosis [4, 44, 46]. Hence, the change in the blood flow by way of a reduction in the perfusion would offer another means to increase the size of the thermally induced lesion.

3.4.5 Modification Through Vascular Occlusion

A starting point of the modification of arterial and portal vein blood flow lies in the occlusion of the vessels prior to RF ablation. The first in vivo experience with modified liver perfusion was made as early as 1998 using internally cooled probes [47]. The blood flow through the hepatic arteries or the portal vein was selectively interrupted using a balloon occlusion. After 12 min of ablation, a coagulation diameter of 2.9 cm was achieved in the case of a portal vein occlusion, in comparison to 2.4 cm by normal flow. In the case of artery occlusion, animal tests showed a coagulation diameter ranging from 2.5 to 2.7 cm. The influence of systematic occlusion of arteries and/or veins has already been examined on patients: two similarly sized colorectal liver metastases (2.2–4.2 cm) in three patients were treated by intraoperative RF ablation [47]. In each patient, one tumor was initially ablated without change to the flow, and subsequently the other tumor was ablated occluding not only the arteries but also the portal vein (similar to the intraoperative Pringle maneuver). The resulting coagulation was significantly larger when using the occlusion (4.1±1.0 cm vs 2.5±0.5 cm).

3.4.6 Modification Through Additive Drugs

In animal tests, Goldberg et al. attempted to influence liver perfusion during RF ablation with internally cooled RF probes using drugs [48]. Blood flow and therefore perfusion were markedly altered using an intra-arterial applied vasopressin or high dose halothane. The thermally induced necrosis produced after intravenous vasopressin had a diameter of 1.3 cm, those after halothane had a diameter of 3.2 cm (vs 2.2 cm in the control group with physiological flow).

3.5 Combined Therapies

One of the most important purposes in the field of tumor RF therapy is to obtain a complete destruction of the pathological tissue in a single procedure. In the case of a liver malignancy larger than 3.5 cm, there is a large risk that the tumor will not be fully destroyed through thermal ablation in a single procedure. Solbiati et al. have reported a relapse rate up to 37% in a long-term study of US-guided RF ablation of liver metastases [17]. However, the imaging modality used (US), and the patient selection in this study (large tumors, synchronous or already surgically treated patients) obviously play a significant role in the relapse rate. Hence, therapy combining transarterial chemoembolization (TACE) with RF ablation can lead to improved clinical results [49], since a sensitization of tumor cells at high temperatures caused by prior damage has been already reported [27]. In the case of hepatocellular carcinomas (HCCs), especially larger than 3.5 cm, a combination of TACE and RF ablation can even result in successful treatment [50]. Furthermore, tests show that larger coagulation can be achieved through previous percutaneous alcohol instillation or a simultaneous application of doxorubicin with RF ablation [51].

3.6 Potential Interactions of Radiofrequency Ablation with the Immune System

As seen above, tumor destruction induced by RF ablation is achieved primarily by local cell coagulation necrosis through tissue heating [24, 29, 51]. This necrotic process is irreversible and still extends to the surrounding cells in the following days or weeks after ablation. Contact with necrotic cells has been shown to induce the maturation of dendritic cells (DCs) into competent antigen-presenting cells [52, 53]. The signals delivered by necrotic cells to DCs are being investigated intensively. Two important components that were recently identified are heat shock proteins (HSPs), such as Hsp70 or Hsp90 [54], which are also induced upon cellular stress, and uric acid [55]. These components have been classified as danger signals, because they are able to alert the immune system by activating antigen-presenting cells (APCs) and inducing T lymphocyte responses to foreign antigens. Indeed, it has been shown that HSPs and uric acid can stimulate an antitumoral CD8+ T cell response in different mouse models [55, 57]. Increased cellular and membrane expression of Hsp70 and Hsp90 has been observed several hours after RF ablation of human liver tumors [58, 59]. Using a specific ELISA, the Hsp70 level in the serum of RF-treated patients was observed before and after RF ablation: results show a transient increase in Hsp70 in several patients 1 day after ablation. This increase was no longer detectable 3 days or several weeks to months afterward [60]. A second approach to understanding the relationship between RF ablation and immunity is to seek T cell activation against the tumor after ablation. This has been done in two animal models. Indeed, a T cell infiltration in the residual tumoral tissue and an activation of antitumor effector T cells were observed [61, 62].

Thus, RF ablation obviously creates a local situation that is suitable for recruiting and activating diverse immune effector cells. In addition to the local destruction of neoplastic tissue, RF ablation may induce an antitumoral activation of the immune system. This effect may constitute an additional beneficial aspect of the RF treatment.

3.7 Optimizing the Radiofrequency Technique

It is not easy to define a specific RF system as the best for percutaneous use, as the many different types of tumors require different RF protocols (ablation probes, ablation length, and applied energy). A recent comparative study of different monopolar devices showed that the largest volume of ablated tissue was obtained with the perfusion electrode, but the coagulation was irregular and unpredictable. The largest mean volume of thermally induced necrosis produced with an acceptable spherical shape was achieved using the cluster electrode [63]. The expandable 12-tine umbrella electrode produced more spherical coagulation but with a slightly more reduced coagulation volume. However, clinical success depends on the skills of the physician, his knowledge in oncology, and both key factors: the imaging used for monitoring as well as the tumor's biological features.

Finally, the use of the imaging procedure to monitor image-guided RF ablation needs to be critically viewed. US limited because of the acoustic shadow and the hyperechoic signal produced by RF ablation, which means that delineating the tumor remains difficult during or immediately after ablation. Repositioning the RF electrode, which is required to treat lesions with a safety margin in a single procedure, may be uncertain since differentiation between already ablated and residual tumor tissue is almost impracticable with US. CT often is not sensitive enough to detect the tumor because of the equilibrium phase. This is especially true if several tumors have to be treated at the same time. The total amount of iodized contrast medium that can be injected is limited, and a differentiation between ablated tissue and surrounding liver parenchyma after treatment may be impossible. RF ablation using MRI appears to be very promising because of its intrinsic excellent soft-tissue contrast, true multiplanar capabilities, and high spatial resolution. In most published studies, closed-bore MR scanners have been used for ablation of brain tumors [64, 65]. Recently several studies have been described with the complete procedure carried out under MR guidance using open-architecture interventional low-field scanners [66–68]. In magnetic resonance tomography, true multiplanar imaging is possible because of the free choice of gradient fields. The imaging plane could always be angulated to optimal orientation showing tumor and RF applicator at once. Completeness of tumor destruction can therefore be evaluated by T2-weighted fast spin-echo sequences immediately after the ablation procedure without using contrast medium. Residual tumor tissue mainly exhibits hyperintense signal compared to hypointense signal of thermocoagulated tissue. This is one major advantage of MR over CT or US guidance, which both need repeated administrations of contrast-medium for sufficient tissue contrast, leading to accumulation of contrast medium within the tissue and subsequent reduction in tumor/coagulation conspicuity. Since the principle of thermal ablation offers the potential for an indefinite number of RF applications at the same time, US and CT therefore have a major disadvantage compared with MR imaging. MR imaging should allow for higher efficiency of complete tumor destruction with fewer ablation sessions as compared to other imaging modalities.

3.8 Conclusion

The aim of image-guided RF ablation for tumor therapy lies in a complete destruction of the tumor tissue with a surrounding margin of nontumorous tissue. This means the development of larger coagulation volume, which can be achieved through a controlled energy deposition, and sufficient imaging allowing ideal targeting of the tumor combined with monitoring of the ablation course. MR imaging is able to provide all requisites for image-guided ablation in a reproducible manner. The ever-increasing technological development of the RF devices will ensure that the procedure will improve in the future, resulting in widespread use of RF in routine clinical practice. RF ablation has shown in various phase II and phase III studies that a safe and effective destruction of tumor tissue is possible, and that patients may benefit from image-guided RF therapy. A further advantage of this minimally invasive therapy lies in the low complication rate of RF ablation. The most suitable tumor pattern for image guided RF ablation must now be defined, as well as the therapies that can be systematically combined with RF, and finally how RF can be integrated into current oncological concepts.

References

1. Gazelle GS, Goldberg SN, Solbiati L, Livraghi T (2002) Tumor ablation with radio-frequency energy. Radiology 217:633–646
2. Wood BJ, Ramkaransingh JR, Fojo T, Walther MM, Libutti SK (2002) Percutaneous tumor ablation with radiofrequency. Cancer 94:443–451
3. Sweet WH, Mark VH, Hamlin H (1960) Radiofrequency lesions in the central nervous system of man and cat, including case reports of eight bulbar pain-tract interruptions. J Neurosurg 17:213–225
4. Solbiati L, Goldberg SN, Ierace T, Livraghi T, Meloni F, Dellanoce M, Sironi S, Gazelle GS (1997) Hepatic metastases: percutaneous radiofrequency ablation with cooled-tip electrodes. Radiology 205:367–373
5. Rossi S, Di Stasi M, Buscarini E, Quaretti P, Garbagnati F, Squassante L, Paties CT, Silverman PE, Buscarini L (1996) Percutaneous RF interstitial thermal ablation in the treatment of hepatic cancer. Am J Roentgenol 169:759–769
6. Livraghi T, Goldberg SN, Lazzaroni S et al. (1999) Small hepatocellular carcinoma: treatment with radio-frequency ablation versus ethanol injection. Radiology 210:655–661
7. Lencioni R, Crocetti L (2005) A critical appraisal of the literature on local ablative therapies for hepatocellular carcinoma. Clin Liver Dis 9:301–314
8. Livraghi T, Solbiati L, Meloni F, Ierace T, Goldberg SN, Gazelle GS (2003) Percutaneous radiofrequency ablation of liver metastases in potential candidates for resection: the test of time approach. Cancer 12:3027–3035
9. Tateishi R, Shiina S, Teratani T et al. (2005) Percutaneous radiofrequency ablation for hepatocellular carcinoma: an analysis of 1000 cases. Cancer 103:1201–1209
10. Vogl T, Mack M, Straub R, Zangos S, Woitaschek, Eichler K, Engelmann K (2001) Thermische Ablation von Lebermetastasen. Der Radiologe 41:49–55
11. Shibata T, Iimuro Y, Yamamoto Y, Maetoni Y, Ametani F, Itoh K, Konishi J (2002) Small hepatocellular carcinoma: comparison of radio-frequency ablation and percutaneous microwave coagulation therapy. Radiology 223:331–337
12. Cline HE, Hynynen K, Watkins RD, Adams WJ, Schenck JF, Ettinger RH, Vetro JP, Jolesz FA (1995) Focussed US system for MR imaging-guided tumor ablation. Radiology 194:31–737
13. Onik GM, Atkinson D, Zemel R, Weaver ML (1993) Cryosurgery of liver cancer. Sem Surg Oncol 9:309–317
14. Silverman SG, Tuncali K, Adams DF, van Sonnenberg E, Zou KH, Kacher DF, Morrison PR, Jolesz FA (2000) MR imaging-guided percutaneous cryotherapy of liver tumors: initial experience. Radiology 217:657–664

15. Rossi S, Buscarini E, Garbagnati F, DiStasi M, Quaretti P, Rago M, Zangrandi A, Andreola S, Silverman D, Buscarini L (1998) Percutaneous treatment of small hepatic tumors by an expandable RF needle electrode. Am J Roentgenol 170:1015–1022
16. Curley SA, Izzo F, Delrio P, Ellis CM, Grandi J, Vallone P, Fiore F, Pignata S, Daniele B, Cremona F (1999) Radiofrequency ablation of unresectable primary and metastatic hepatic malignancies: results in 123 patients. Ann Surg 1230:1–8
17. Solbiati L, Livraghi T, Goldberg SN, Ierace T, Meloni F, Dellanoce M, Cova L, Halpern E, Gazelle GS (2001) Percutaneous radio-frequency ablation of hepatic metastases from colorectal cancer: long-term results in 117 patients. Radiology 221:159–166
18. D'Arsonval MA (1891) Action physiologique des courants alternatifs. CR Soc Biol 43:283–286
19. Organ LW (1976) Electrophysiologic principles of radiofrequency lesion making. Appl Neurophysiol 39:69–76
20. McGahan JP, Brock JM, Tesluk H, Gu WZ, Schneider P, Browning PD (1992) Hepatic ablation with use of radiofrequency electrocautery in the animal model. J Vasc Interv Radiol 3:291–297
21. Zervas NT, Kuwayama A (1972) Pathological characteristics of experimental thermal lesions: comparison of induction heating and radiofrequency electrocoagulation. J Neurosurg 37:418–422
22. Goldberg SN, Gazelle GS, Dawson SL, Rittman WJ, Mueller PR, Rosenthal DI (1995) Tissue ablation with radiofrequency: effect of probe size, gauge, duration and temperature on lesion volume. Acad Radiol 2:399–404
23. Trübenbach J, Pereira PL, Schick F, Claussen CD, Huppert PE (1998) MRI-guided radiofrequency ablation of liver tumors: a valuable and minimally-invasive therapeutic option. Min Invas Ther 6:533–539
24. Goldberg SN, Gazelle GS, Compton CC, Mueller PR, Tanabe KK (2000) Treatment of intrahepatic malignancy with radiofrequency ablation: radiologic–pathologic correlation. Cancer 88:2452–2463
25. Pennes HH (1948) Analysis of tissue and arterial blood temperatures in the resting human forearm. J Appl Physiol 1:93–122
26. Hill RP, Hunt JW (1987) Hyperthermia. In: Tannock IF, Hill RP (eds) The basic science of oncology. Pergamon New York, pp 337–357
27. Seegenschmidt MH, Brady LW, Sauer R (1990) Interstitial thermoradiotherapy: review on technical and clinical aspects. Am J Clin Oncol 13:352–363
28. Larson TR, Bostwick DG, Corcia A (1996) Temperature-correlated histopathologic changes following microwave thermoablation of obstructive tissue in patients with benign prostatic hyperplasia. Urology 47:463–469
29. Thomsen S (1991) Pathologic analysis of photothermal and photomechanical effects of laser-tissue interactions. Photochem Photobiol 53:825–835
30. Goldberg SN, Solbiati L, Hahn PF, Cosman E, Conrad JE, Fogle R, Gazelle GS (1998) Large-volume tissue ablation with radiofrequency by using a clustered, internally-cooled electrode technique: laboratory and clinical experience in liver metastases. Radiology 209:371–379
31. Trübenbach J, Huppert PE, Pereira PL, Ruck P, Claussen CD (1997) Radiofrequenzablation der Leber in vitro: Effektivitätserhöhung mittels perfundierter Sonden. Fortschr Röntgenstr 167:633–637
32. Goldberg SN, Gazelle GS (2001) Radiofrequency tissue ablation: physical principles and techniques for increasing coagulation necrosis. Hepatogastroenterol 48:359–367
33. Goldberg SN, Gazelle GS, Dawson SL, Mueller PR, Rittman WJ, Rosenthal DI (1995) Radiofrequency tissue ablation using multiprobe arrays: greater tissue destruction than multiple probes operating alone. Acad Radiol 2:670–674
34. LeVeen RF (1997) Laser hyperthermia and radiofrequency ablation of hepatic lesions. Semin Int Radiology 14:313–324
35. Goldberg SN, Gazelle GS, Solbiati L, Rittman WJ, Mueller PR (1996) Radiofrequency tissue ablation: increased lesion diameter with a perfusion electrode. Acad Radiol 3:636–644
36. Lorentzen T (1996) A cooled needle electrode for radiofrequency tissue ablation: Thermodynamic aspects of improved performance compared with conventional needle design. Acad Radiol 13:556–563

37. Schmidt D, Trübenbach J, König CW, Putzhammer H, Duda SH, Claussen CD, Pereira PL (2003) Automated saline-enhanced radiofrequency thermal ablation: initial results in ex-vivo liver. Am J Roentgenol 180:163–165
38. Kettenbach J, Peer K, Grurin M, Berger J, Hupfl M, Lammer J (2001) MRI-guided percutaneous radiofrequency ablation of neoplasms using a MR-compatible RF-system: first technical and clinical experiences (abstract). Radiology 221:626
39. Tacke J, Mahnken A, Roggan A, Günther RW (2004) Multipolar radiofrequency ablation: first clinical results. Fortschr Röntgenstr 176:324–329
40. McGahan JP, Wei-Zhong G, Brock JM, Tesluk H, Jones CD (1996) Hepatic ablation using bipolar radiofrequency electrocautery. Acad Radiol 3:418–422
41. Burdio F, Guemes A, Burdio JM, Navarro A, Sousa R, Castiella T, Cruz I, Burzaco O, Lozano R (2003) Bipolar saline-enhanced electrode for radiofrequency ablation: results of experimental study of in vivo porcine liver. Radiology 229:447–456
42. Goldberg SN, Stein M, Gazelle GS, Sheiman RG, Kruskal JB, Clouse ME (1999) Percutaneous radiofrequency tissue ablation: optimization of pulsed-RF technique to increase coagulation necrosis. J Vasc Interv Radiol 10:907–916
43. Merkle E, Goldberg SN, Boll DT, Shankaranarayanan A, Boaz T, Jacobs GH, Wendt M, Lewin JS (1999) Effect of superparamagnetic MR contrast agents on radiofrequency-induced temperature distribution: in vitro measurements in polyacrylamide phantoms and in-vivo results in a rabbit liver model. Radiology 212:459–466
44. Melvyn Lobo S, Afzal KS, Ahmed M, Kruskal JB, Lenkinski RE, Goldberg SN (2004) Radiofrequency ablation: modelling the enhanced temperature response to adjuvant NaCl pre-treatment. Radiology 230:175–182
45. Goldberg SN, Solbiati L, Halpern EF, Gazelle GS (2000) Variables affecting proper system grounding for radiofrequency ablation in animal model. J Vasc Interv Radiol 11:1069–1075
46. Debaere T, Denys A, Wood BJ, Lassau N, Kardache M, Vilgrain V, Menu Y, Roche A (2001) Radiofrequency liver ablation: experimental comparative study of water-cooled versus expandable systems. Am J Roentgenol 176:187–192
47. Goldberg SN, Hahn PF, Tanabe KK, Mueller PR, Schima W, Athanasoutis CA, Compton CC, Solbiati L, Gazelle GS (1998) Percutaneous radiofrequency tissue ablation: does perfusion-mediated tissue cooling limit coagulation necrosis? J Vasc Interv Radiol 9:101–111
48. Goldberg SN, Hahn PF, Halpern E, Fogle R, Gazelle GS (1998) Radiofrequency tissue ablation: effect of pharmacologic modulation of blood flow on coagulation diameter. Radiology 209:761–769
49. Buscarini L, Buscarini E, diStasi M, Quaretti P, Zangrandi A (1999) Percutaneous radiofrequency thermal ablation combined with transcatheter arterial embolization in the treatment of large hepatocellular carcinoma. Ultraschall Med 20:47–53
50. Akamatsu M, Yoshida H, Obi S, Sato S, Koike Y, Fujishima T, Tateishi R, Imamura M, Hamamura K, Teratani T, Shina S, Ishikawa T, Omata M (2004) Evaluation of transcatheter arterial embolization prior to percutaneous tumor ablation in patients with hepatocellular carcinoma: a randomized controlled trial. Liver Int 24:625–629
51. Goldberg SN, Saldinger PF, Gazelle GS, Huertas JL, Stuart KE, Jacobs T, Kruskal JB (2001) Percutaneous tumor ablation: increased coagulation necrosis with combined radiofrequency and percutaneous doxorubicin injection. Radiology 220:420–427
52. Itoh T, Orba Y, Takei H, Ishida Y, Saitoh M, Nakamura H, Meguro T, Horita S, Fujita M, Nagashima K (2002) Immunohistochemical detection of hepatocellular carcinoma in the setting of ongoing necrosis after radiofrequency ablation. Mod Pathol 15:110–115
53. Sauter B, Albert ML, Fransisco L, Larsson M, Somersan S, Bhardwaj N (2000) Consequences of cell death: exposure to necrotic tumor cells, but not primary tissue cells or apoptotic cells, induces maturation of immunostimulatory dendritic cells. J Exp Med 191:423–434
54. Basu S, Binder RJ, Suto R, Anderson KM, Srivastava PK (2000) Necrotic but not apoptotic cell death releases heat shock proteins, which deliver a partial maturation signal to dendritic cells and activate the NF-kappa B pathway. Int Immunol 12:1539–1546
55. Shi Y, Evans JE, Rock KL (2003) Molecular identification of a danger signal that alerts the immune system to dying cells. Nature 425:516–521

56. Hu DE, Moore AM, Thomsen LL, Brindle KM (2004) Uric acid promotes tumor immune rejection. Cancer Res 64:5059–5062
57. Srivastava P (2002) Interaction of heat shock proteins with peptides and antigen presenting cells: chaperoning of the innate and adaptive immune responses. Annu Rev Immunol 20:395–425
58. Schueller G, Kettenbach J, Sedivy R, Stift A, Friedl J, Gnant M, Lammer J (2004) Heat shock protein expression induced by percutaneous radiofrequency ablation of hepatocellular carcinoma in vivo. Int J Oncol 24:609–613
59. Yang WL, Nair DG, Makizumi R, Gallos G, Ye X, Sharma RR, Ravikumar TS (2004) Heat shock protein 70 is induced in mouse human colon tumor xenografts after sublethal radiofrequency ablation. Ann Surg Oncol 11:399–406
60. Zerbini Z, Pilli M, Penna A, Pelosi G, Schianchi C, Molinari A, Schivazappa S, Zibera C, Fagnoni FF, Ferrari C, Missale G (2006) Radiofrequency thermal ablation of hepatocellular carcinoma liver nodules can activate and enhance tumor-specific T-cell responses. Cancer Res 66:1139–1146
61. Wissniowski TT, Hansler J, Neureiter D, Frieser M, Schaber S, Esslinger B, Voll R, Strobel D, Hahn EG, Schuppan D (2003) Activation of tumor-specific T lymphocytes by radio-frequency ablation of the VX2 hepatoma in rabbits. Cancer Res 63:6496–6500
62. Den Brok MH, Sutmuller RP, van der Voort R, Bennink EJ, Figdor CG, Ruers TJ, Adema GJ (2004) In situ tumor ablation creates an antigen source for the generation of antitumor immunity. Cancer Res 64:4024–4029
63. Pereira PL, Trübenbach J, Schenk M, Subke J, Kröber S, Schäfer I, Remy CT, Schmidt D, Brieger J, Claussen CD (2004) Radiofrequency ablation: in vivo comparison of four commercially available devices in pig livers. Radiology 232:482–490
64. Kahn T, Bettag M, Ulrich F et al. (1994) MRI-guided laser-induced interstitial thermotherapy of cerebral neoplasms. J Comput Assist Tomogr 18:519–532
65. Anzai Y, Lufkin R, DeSalles A, Hamilton DR, Farahani K, Black KL (1995) Preliminary experience with MR-guided thermal ablation of brain tumors. AJNR Am J Neuroradiol 16:39–52
66. Lewin JS, Connell CF, Duerk JL et al. (1998) Interactive MRI-guided radiofrequency interstitial thermal ablation of abdominal tumors: clinical trial for evaluation of safety and feasibility. J Magn Reson Imaging 8:40–47
67. Reither K, Wacker F, Ritz JP et al. (2000) Laser-induced thermotherapy (LITT) for liver metastasis in an open 0.2T MRI. Rofo Fortschr Geb Rontgenstr Neuen Bildgeb Verfahr 172:175–178
68. Lewin JS, Nour SG, Connell CF, Sulman A, Duerk JL, Resnick MI, Haaga JR (2004) Phase II trial of interactive MR imaging-guided interstitial radiofrequency thermal ablation of primary kidney tumors: initial experience. Radiology 232:835–845

The Surgical Approach for Radiofrequency Ablation of Liver Tumors

Guido Schumacher, Robert Eisele, Antonino Spinelli, Peter Neuhaus

4.1 Introduction

Before deciding to perform a surgical radiofrequency ablation (RFA), it must be clear that a RFA is the correct treatment modality for a liver tumor of a particular patient. An interdisciplinary meeting, which consists of surgeons, radiologists, and gastroenterologists, or medical oncologists should decide individually which patients receive surgical resection, liver transplantation, RFA, other treatment modalities, or whether two or more of these options may be combined. When the tumor or tumors are considered to be unresectable, and the conference has chosen RFA as the best alternative treatment option, the decision must be made as to whether the percutaneous, laparoscopic, or open surgical approach is appropriate in a particular patient. Here we discuss surgical RFA and compare the advantages, disadvantages, and technical aspects.

4.2 Surgical Treatment or Radiofrequency Ablation

Liver resection for colorectal metastases seems to provide long-term survival with a 5-year survival of 25%–40% (Fong et al. 1997; Scheele et al. 1995). Neoadjuvant chemotherapy may even improve resectability. Thirteen to 16% of unresectable tumors could be rendered resectable (Leonard et al. 2005). The most important factor is to achieve a R0 status after resection. Liver resection of metastases from other primary tumors such as breast, stomach, pancreas, melanoma, or others must be decided individually when the liver is the only tumor site in those patients. Resection seems to benefit these patients (Bentrem et al. 2005). Primary liver cancer, which is mainly hepatocellular carcinoma (HCC) or cholangiocarcinoma (CCC), is a particular cancer type because HCC arises in the underlying liver cirrhosis in 90%, which limits resectability. Furthermore, liver transplantation (LTX) for both HCC and CCC is a therapeutic option. LTX for HCC is the therapy with the best long-term survival of 71% after 5 years (Jonas et al. 2001). CCC in general is not a good indication for LTX. However, there is a highly selective group in which LTX may be favorable over other therapies (Pascher et al. 2003).

The decision to undertake a RFA can be made when contraindications will not allow surgical resection. In these cases, a RFA may be considered as the next treatment option of choice. Indications for RFA are listed in Table 4.1. Like liver resection, the primary goal after RFA is to achieve a tumor-free situation. There is no benefit when the ablation is incomplete (Siperstein et al. 2000).

When the decision is made to perform a radiofrequency ablation, the first approach to consider is percutaneous, which is easy to perform when the tumor is clearly visible in ultrasound, CT, or MRI scan. Furthermore, the tumor should not be on the liver surface because of the possible injury of organs such as colon, duodenum, gall bladder, kidney, adrenal gland, diaphragm, stomach, and heart. If a percutaneous RFA is not possible for different reasons, the surgeon will decide whether a laparoscopic or an open surgical approach would be beneficial in the individual situation.

Table 4.1 Indications for radiofrequency ablation (RFA)

HCC	Metastases
Irresectable (cirrhosis)	Inoperable tumors
No indication for transplantation	Small central tumors
Patient on the waiting list for LTX	Synchronous metastases
Patient refuses surgery	Patient refuses surgery
Underlying or accompanying disease	Underlying or accompanying disease
Tumor recurrence	Combination of RFA and resection

HCC, hepatocellular carcinoma

Table 4.2 Contraindications for percutaneous radiofrequency ablation

Tumors on the liver surface
Insufficient visibility of the tumor
Surgery is required (cholecystectomy)
Difficult access to the tumor
Intraoperative ultrasound is desired

Table 4.3 Organs of potential injury during radiofrequency ablation

Gallbladder
Duodenum
Colon
Stomach
Right kidney
Right adrenal gland
Diaphragm
Heart

4.2.1 Indications for Surgical Radiofrequency Ablation

In general, the indication for a surgical approach is given when a percutaneous approach is not indicated, since all difficulties that are faced during percutaneous RFA can be avoided by surgery. Table 4.2 shows the contraindications for a percutaneous RFA, the most important of which is the tumor on the liver surface. There are reports on the instillation of saline in the space between the liver surface with the tumor and the adjacent organ to keep the adjacent organs at a certain distance to avoid injury (Kapoor and Hunter 2003). However, in our opinion, protection cannot be achieved without a remaining risk of injury. A particular situation is found when tumor recurrences manifest on the resection surface. Strong adhesions of adjacent organs with the liver surface from previous surgery will cause a very high risk of injury during percutaneous RFA. Injection of saline cannot remove adjacent organs from that surface. This situation has to be considered as absolute contraindication for percutaneous RFA. The organs most likely affected are stomach, duodenum, and greater omentum after left-side liver resection and colon, duodenum, and small intestine after right-side liver resection (Table 4.3). The visibility of the tumor before starting the RFA is crucial. For the percutaneous approach, ultrasound does not always allow visualization of the tumor. In this situation, RFA should be CT- or MR-guided, or using a surgical approach, either laparoscopically or through open surgery, which may ensure a safe ablation. When additional surgery is required, a surgical approach for RFA should be done in combination with the other surgery. Most frequently, a cholecystectomy will be needed. We always perform a cholecystectomy when the tumor is located in proximity to the gallbladder. Other

Table 4.4 Indications for surgical radiofrequency ablation

Intraoperative ultrasound with the possible detection of additional tumor nodules
Safe ablation on liver surface
Reduced flow of the portal vein during pneumoperitoneum or Pringle maneuver
Combination with other surgical interventions (cholecystectomy or others)
Combination with liver resection
Safe and precise placement of the electrode into the tumor
When intraoperative ultrasound is required to detect additional tumor nodules

surgeries that can be performed during RFA are liver resection, biopsies from peritoneum or lymph nodes, or adhesiolysis. When the tumor is not easily accessible because of an uncomfortable location, for example in segment VIII on the liver dome, a surgical approach may also be discussed to achieve a safer placement of the RFA electrode. For better visibility and intraoperative tumor staging, an intraoperative ultrasound may be desired, which should also lead to the decision to perform a surgical approach, either laparoscopic or through open surgery.

Besides the contraindications for a percutaneous RFA, which lead to the surgical RFA, there are also direct indications which favor the surgical approach of RFA, as shown in Table 4.4.

Intraoperative ultrasound may detect additional tumor nodules in almost 30% of all patients (Kokudo et al. 1996). Thus, intraoperative ultrasound helps to achieve an R0 situation in 30% of the patients who would remain inapparent otherwise. Therefore we perform a thorough ultrasound examination of all liver areas during surgical RFA. During laparotomy, palpation of the liver, especially in soft metastatic livers with hard tumor nodules, gives additional valuable information on the tumor burden. When tumors are located on the liver surface, we always perform surgical RFA. Under optical guidance, an ablation under safe protection of adjacent organs is technically easy and recommended. Furthermore, reduction of the blood flow may help to increase the ablation zone either by reducing the flow of the portal vein during pneumoperitoneum, as shown before, or by using a Pringle maneuver during open surgery. This maneuver should be used when tumors have direct contact with large vessels. The Pringle maneuver reduces the heat-sink effect, which is a cooling effect of the blood inside the vessel. The placement of the electrode is most accurate during open surgery. The electrode may be placed less accurately during laparoscopic RFA when the tumor does not allow easy access. In these situations, an open surgical approach will abolish such difficulties by allowing the liver to be mobilized and providing greater variability for the needle tract.

4.2.2 Laparoscopic or Open Surgical Radiofrequency Ablation

The surgical team must decide whether the surgical approach should be laparoscopic or open through laparotomy. Studies indicate that both the laparoscopic and the open surgical approach have similar results in tumor control. However, the proportion of round/ovoid lesions (20% vs 64%) was lower ($p = 0.043$) and warm-up time (20.2 ± 14.0 vs 10.7 ± 7.5) was longer ($p = 0.049$) for the laparoscopic than for the open groups, respectively (Scott et al. 2001). Several factors favor the laparoscopic approach, as shown in Table 4.5. There is experimental data and clini-

Table 4.5 Advantages of laparoscopic over open surgical radiofrequency ablation

Minimally invasive
Reduced flow of the portal vein during pneumoperitoneum
Exploration of the whole abdominal cavity
Short hospital stay

cal indication that the pneumoperitoneum decreases the flow of the portal vein, which leads to an increased ablation site (Smith et al. 2004). It appears to be a safe method to ablate HCC nodules (Montorsi et al. 2001). A major advantage of the laparoscopic approach is the lower invasiveness of the intervention. Patient comfort is much higher because of less pain, faster recovery, and low morbidity after treatment of otherwise untreatable tumors. Intraoperative ultrasound is mandatory for laparoscopic RFA to visualize the tumors. The use of the ultrasound probe is expensive and technically demanding. When liver metastases are treated, the ultrasound probe has full contact to the liver surface because the liver parenchyma is soft. In the case of liver cirrhosis, the liver is hard and mostly it presents a surface with large and small regeneration nodules, which causes loss of contact of the ultrasound probe with the liver. Not all disadvantages of the percutaneous approach for RFA can be avoided using the laparoscopic approach. Much better and safer placement of the RFA electrode is possible using the open surgical approach. Once the abdominal cavity is opened, the liver is technically easy to explore using palpation and intraoperative ultrasound. Not only are the areas of the liver surface easy to explore, but also areas on the back side of the liver when the liver is mobilized. The consequence of the easy handling is a safer placement of the electrode during open surgery compared to laparoscopic approach. This is most important for cirrhotic livers. In our department, we performed RFA for HCC in over 90% of the patients, in which 80% suffered from liver cirrhosis. Thus, we perform mostly an open surgical RFA in patients with liver cirrhosis, unless the tumor is easily accessible with the laparoscopic or percutaneous approach. Many patients suffer from recurrent disease after surgery, or had previous surgery such as colon or rectum resection. These patients present with intra-abdominal adhesions, which may be too extensive to perform a risk-free laparoscopy. In such patients, we always perform an open surgical RFA when the percutaneous approach is not suitable for this particular patient. Removing adhesions during open surgery is safe and complete. In addition to the improved intra-abdominal exploration using the open surgical approach, a lymphadenectomy in the liver hilum and coeliac trunk can be performed safely, which gives important staging information. As mentioned for the laparoscopic RFA, a reduction of the blood flow to the liver results in a decrease in the heat sink effect and an increase of the ablation zone. During open surgery, an occlusion of the entire hepatoduodenal ligament, which includes hepatic artery and portal vein (Pringle maneuver), reduces the blood flow completely. An increased ablation area is assumed by reduction of the heat sink effect (Scott et al. 2002; Wiersinga 2003). However, an experimental study in pigs showed that there is no increase in the ablation site even when the tumor is located next to large vessels (Shen et al. 2003). More studies are needed to elucidate completely the benefit of the Pringle maneuver. Many patients present with multiple tumor nodules in both liver lobes. Individually, the surgical treatment of these tumors may be a liver resection, an RFA, or the combination of both. In cirrhotic livers, large liver resections are not possible because too much functional liver tissue is lost. Resection of smaller parts of the liver such as segmentectomies or wedge resections may be possible, but in the case of a tumor that requires large liver resections such as hemihepatectomy, the indication for liver resection should be decided in a center with great experience in liver surgery. With multifocal tumors in cirrhotic livers, only small resections may be possible. Either small resections, RFA, or the combination of both may be suitable. When patients present with liver metastases in a normal liver, liver resection may be more extended and still be combined with RFA. Deciding on the correct treatment modality should be done individually by experienced liver surgeons. Extended liver resection is mostly possible because of normal liver function. Additional nodules may be either resected by wedge resection or treated with RFA. The advantages of the open surgical approach over the laparoscopic approach are summarized in Table 4.6.

In addition to the advantages of one technique over the other, the disadvantages faced during each technique must be weighed. In Table 4.7 the disadvantages of the laparoscopic over the open surgical approach are listed.

However, the open surgical approach also has disadvantages over the laparoscopic approach, as shown in Table 4.8. Surgical resection may cause tumor cell shedding by manipulation of the tu-

Table 4.6 Advantages of open surgery over laparoscopic radiofrequency ablation

Technically easy and access to all parts of the liver
Safest ablation because of most precise placement of the electrode in the tumor
Thorough intraoperative ultrasound to detect additional tumor nodules
Removal of adhesions from previous surgery
Combination with liver resection or other major surgeries
Technically easy Pringle maneuver

Table 4.7 Disadvantages of laparoscopic over open surgical radiofrequency ablation

Technically demanding
The placement of the electrode is less accurate
A laparoscopic ultrasound probe is required
Difficult access to certain areas of the liver
Not possible with severe adhesions from previous surgery
No combination with liver resection or other major surgeries
Pringle maneuver is technically more difficult

mor, which is a factor in disease recurrence. A sequential treatment with RFA and hepatic resection showed that the local recurrence rate may be reduced. However, three out of seven patients developed pulmonary metastases, which possibly occurred through a transvenous migration of tumor cells (Hoffman et al. 2002). More studies are needed to obtain conclusive results on this question.

The recovery after open surgery is longer than after laparoscopy or percutaneous RFA. While all patients had an overnight stay in our department after percutaneous or laparoscopic RFA, the patients after laparotomy with open surgical RFA without liver resection, were hospitalized a minimum of 5 days. There were extensions of the stay in case of temporary liver failure in patients with liver cirrhosis. When RFA was combined with liver resection, the length of the hospitalization was determined by the extent of the liver resection and the liver function. Many patients present with underlying or accompanying disease. After examination of the major organ functions such as heart and lung, the patient may be judged to be too sick for extended surgery. In these patients, we perform a RFA when the tumor is not larger than 3 cm.

In spite of the apparently clear indication for a particular approach, the decision must be made individually.

4.3 Diagnostics

The diagnosis is mainly made with a CT or MRI scan. Besides identification of tumors, this diag-

Table 4.8 Disadvantages of open surgical over laparoscopic radiofrequency ablation

Long recovery from large laparotomy
Underlying or accompanying diseases may limit this approach
Most expensive procedure
Tumor cell shedding

nosis gives information on the size of the liver and parts of the liver such as left lateral liver segments. It is important to estimate the remnant liver portion when extended liver surgery is required. Furthermore, an estimation of the presence of liver cirrhosis is possible by direct signs of liver cirrhosis with increased density of the liver parenchyma or a rough liver surface. Indirect signs of liver cirrhosis may be an increased size of the spleen as a sign for hypersplenism, a hypertrophy of the caudate lobe, identification of collateral veins in case of portal hypertension, or the presence of ascites. Large tumors may cause a thrombosis of the entire portal vein or its branches or of the liver arteries. A preoperative ultrasound is mandatory. If the tumors are visible with a preoperative ultrasound, the operation can be planned with more accuracy. If the tumor is not visible in a preoperative ultrasound, the tumor has to be localized during surgery using intraoperative ultrasound. Since the localization of the tumor is known from the preoperative CT or MRI scan, the tumor may be found easily during intraoperative ultrasound. Regular blood values including transaminases, bilirubin, protein, and albumin levels, platelets, clotting factors, and tumor markers give information about the liver function and stage of cirrhosis. When an HCC is suspected, alpha feto protein (AFP) gives sufficient information. In the case of a cholangiocarcinoma, Ca 19-9 is the marker of choice. In the case of liver metastases, the tumor marker depends on the primary tumor, and should be determined according to this. For colorectal cancer, the most frequently elevated markers are CEA, Ca 19-9, and Ca 72-4.

4.4 Therapy

4.4.1 General Technical Considerations

Before ablation of liver tumors, an estimation of the percentage of liver parenchyma that will be destroyed must be made. In cirrhotic livers, there will be a limitation of the ablation quantity to decrease the risk of postinterventional liver failure. The decision of the approach and the extent of resection or ablation has to be made individually. All patients who present with liver tumors should be evaluated by experienced liver surgeons for possible liver resection. Only when the tumor is considered to be unresectable do the patients move to the next treatment modality, which may be RFA in cases of small tumors. Therefore, all patients with liver tumors should be treated in a center with vast experience with liver tumors. If the total volume of the ablated liver parenchyma is estimated to be to too large, the tumors should be treated in several procedures with a time interval to allow the normal liver parenchyma and the patient to recover. When several tumors are ablated during one procedure, it is recommended to ablate first the tumors in the deeper areas of the livers, because the rising gas bubbles during RFA cause an echogenic area that covers the tumor volume and the deeper areas of the liver.

4.4.2 Laparoscopic Technique

A normal periumbilical incision is made and a pneumoperitoneum with CO_2 is created with an intra-abdominal pressure of 15 mm Hg. A camera is inserted through a 10-mm trocar, and a laparoscopy of the whole abdominal cavity is performed. A second trocar of 12 mm is inserted according to the tumor location. The location has to allow the insertion of a laparoscopic ultrasound probe, which is then able to examine the complete liver. The tract has to be chosen carefully because the RFA electrode should ideally be inserted close to the ultrasound probe. If the ultrasound probe and RFA electrode are inserted in parallel, it is technically easy to follow the electrode during placement and ablation in real-time ultrasound. Sometimes, the location of the tumor does not allow parallel insertion. When the ultrasound probe and the RFA electrode can not be inserted in parallel, the ultrasound probe has to be moved during placement of the RFA electrode to ensure the correct placement. Figure 4.1 shows a typical setup during a laparoscopic RFA. The camera, the laparoscopic ultrasound probe, and the RFA electrode are inserted. In the background, the laparoscopic view of the liver surface on one side and the laparoscopic ultrasound view on the other side is visible on monitors. Figure 4.2 illustrates the relation of the RFA electrode and ultrasound probe in a situation where a parallel placement was not possible. Most often, the trocar for the ultrasound probe is located in the midline of the epigastrium, or in the right upper part of the abdominal wall. After a complete and thorough examination of the liver, the electrode has to be placed under ultrasound guidance. From the practical risk-avoiding point of view, the needle tract should not pass through major blood vessels or bile ducts, which can easily be identified with ultrasound. Furthermore, the direction of the needle tract should not point on important structures or organs such as the liver hilum, heart, etc. In case of an accidental move of the patient or other unpredictable events, the electrode could cause severe damage. When tumors on the liver surface are ablated, the needle tract should not puncture the tumor directly, but should pass through healthy liver tissue before it reaches the tumor to minimize tumor cell seeding. It may be necessary to puncture the tumor directly. In this situation, the electrodes should be deployed before reaching the tumor. After touching the tumor, the electrodes should be deployed further to the desired extent. Figure 4.3 shows a projecting tumor in a segment of a cirrhotic liver (Fig. 4.3a). A needle tract through nontumorous liver tissue cannot ensure a safe placement of the electrode. After deployment of the electrode to a certain degree, the single electrodes were pushed into the tumor under ultrasound guidance, and the ablation process was initiated (Fig. 4.3b). After completion of the ablation, the tumor changes color, with obvious necrotic areas as indication of necrosis (Fig. 4.3c). Some areas of the liver are still technically difficult to reach with the RFA electrode such as the liver dome of segments VII and VIII of the right liver lobe. After visualizing the tumor with the laparoscopic ultrasound, the percutaneous insertion of the electrode may pass through the lung or the recessus, which may cause pneumothorax. In case of a tumor location with close or direct proximity to the gallbladder, a regular laparoscopic cholecystectomy is performed using resorbable clips for the cystic duct and the cystic artery. If a liver biopsy is desired, it is done under visual guidance with a laparoscopic biopsy forceps, and the bleeding is controlled with bipolar coagulation.

The requirements described for the needle tract limit the variability of its placement, which may impair the safe placement of the electrode. Therefore, the procedure must be planned with caution, and the open surgical approach must always be taken into consideration.

After correct placement of the electrode, the ablation will be started according to the tumor size and the ablation protocol of the particular electrode. In case of apparent incomplete ablation, a replacement after track ablation has to be done to increase the efficiency of the procedure. During ablation, adjacent organs have to be protected with retractors, which are inserted through an additional 5-mm trocar. After removal of the electrode, the puncture site is controlled for eventual bleeding, which may be stopped with bipolar coagulation. A final check of the abdominal cavity is done, and the trocars are removed under visual guidance.

4.4.3 Open Surgical Technique

When RFA is performed as single treatment, an epigastric midline incision is sufficient to treat tumors in the left lateral liver segments. When the tumor is located in segment I, IV, or in the right liver lobe, we prefer the epigastric midline incision with extension to the right side as right transverse laparotomy to obtain an L-shaped incision. After inserting the retractors, a thorough bimanual and ultrasound examination of the entire liver is easily performed. Livers harboring metastases are usually soft, while HCCs mostly grow in hard cirrhotic livers. When liver metastases are ablated, a thorough palpation combined with intraoperative ultrasound gives a reliable estimation of the final tumor burden. Palpation of livers with advanced cirrhosis gives information on tumor burden only when the tumor is located on the liver surface. When number, size, and location of the tumors can be confirmed from the preoperative CT or MRI scans, or when additional tumor nodules are discovered by intraoperative ultrasound, the ablation can be planned. We mobilize the liver when it helps to obtain better access to the tumors. In general, mobilizing the right liver lobe greatly improves the access to all liver tumors of the right liver lobe. Furthermore, this maneuver can remove tumors from direct contact to the vena cava. This increases the efficiency by abolishing the heat-sink effect. When tumors have direct or close contact to the gallbladder, we perform a cholecystectomy. When tumors are located in segment II close to the diaphragm, we divide the left triangular ligament to keep the ablation site distant from the diaphragm and heart. The mobilization of the liver lobes also helps increase the variability of the needle tract, which has importance for different reasons, as mentioned before. After mobilizing the liver, the puncture of large vessels or bile ducts can be avoided. If the needle tract has to point toward structures such as the heart, stomach, colon, duodenum, gall bladder, kidney, adrenal gland, diaphragm, and liver hilum, a surgical towel may be placed between electrode and the structure to be protected. We perform a Pringle maneuver when tumors are located in direct contact with large vessels, especially branches of the portal vein. This will decrease the blood flow and the heat sink effect.

In some patients, the decision for RFA is made only intraoperatively. The tumor appeared to be resectable preoperatively after evaluation of the CT or MRI scans. If the cirrhosis appears to be more advanced than previously estimated, a resection should not be performed. Extended

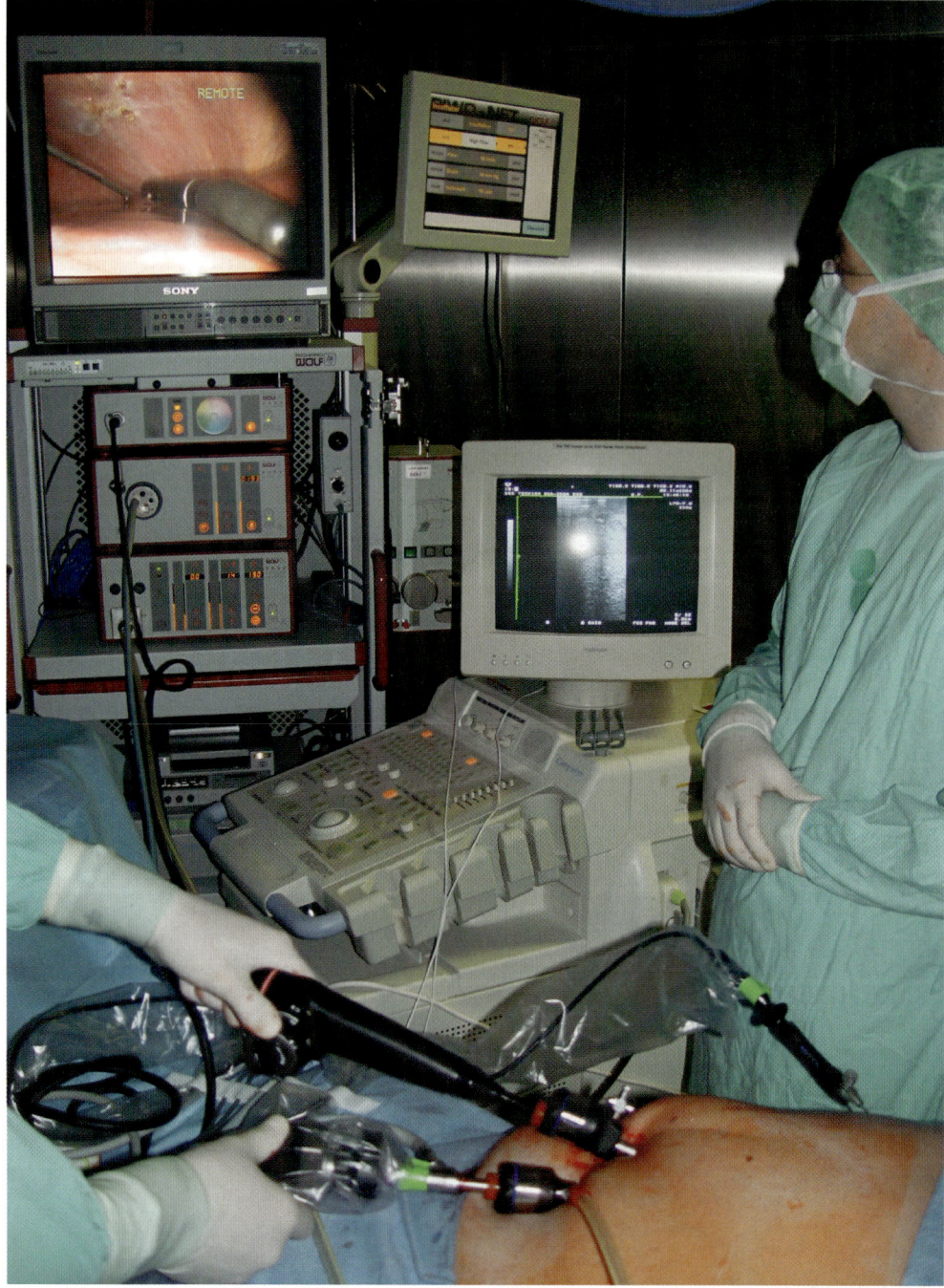

Fig. 4.1 Intraoperative setup during laparoscopic RFA. The camera is inserted through a periumbilical incision; the laparoscopic ultrasound probe is inserted through an epigastric trocar. The RFA electrode is inserted percutaneously under laparoscopic and ultrasound guidance

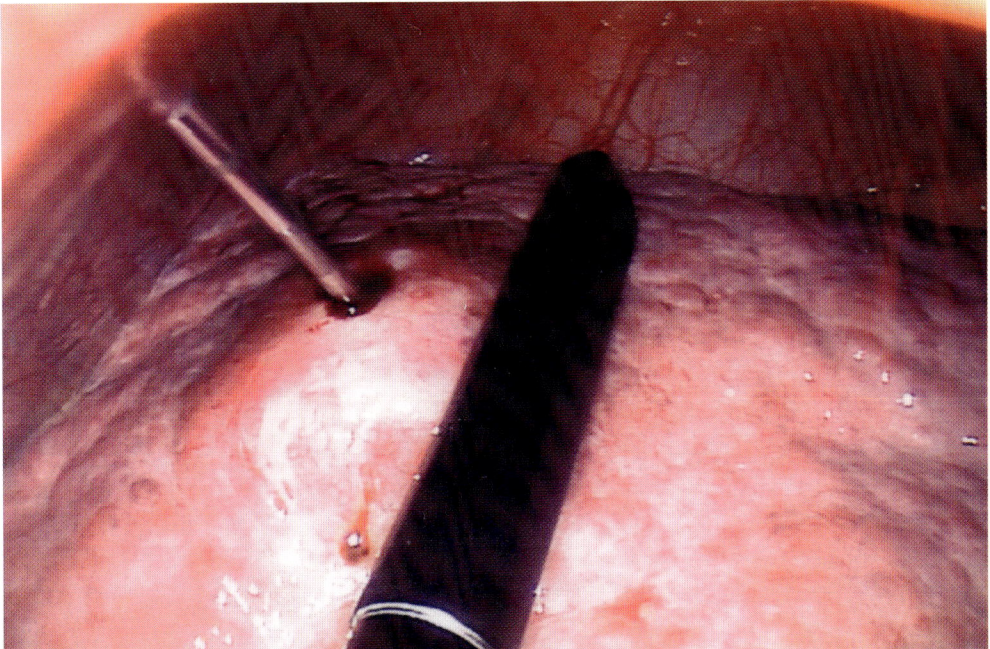

Fig. 4.2 Laparoscopic view of an ultrasound-guided RFA

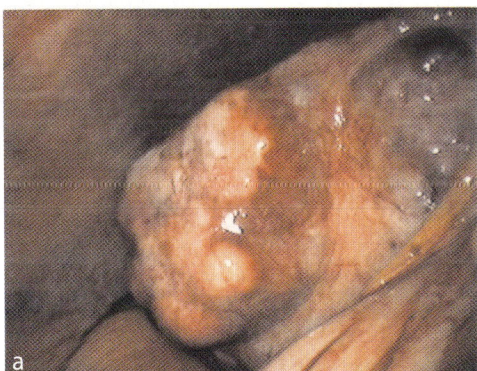

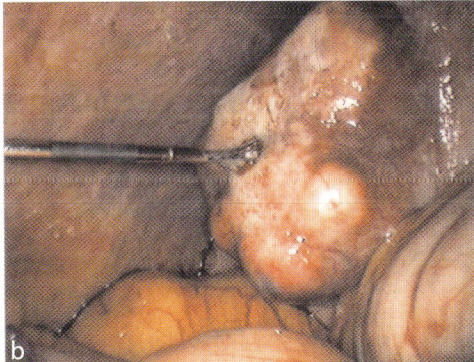

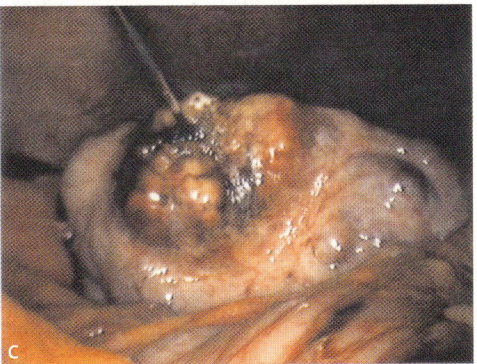

Fig. 4.3a–c Laparoscopic view of an ablation of a protruding HCC in cirrhosis in segment VI. The right colon flexure is removed by a retractor. The color is changed during ablation, indicating the development of complete tumor necrosis. **a** Tumor before ablation. **b** Tumor during ablation. **c** Tumor at the end of ablation

experience is needed to estimate whether resection is possible or not. Factors that favor RFA instead of resection are portal hypertension with hypersplenism, ascites, small remnant liver parenchyma, and the intraoperative aspect of the liver with advanced cirrhosis, even with normal lab values. Livers with Child B or Child C cirrhosis are usually excluded from surgery with only a few exceptions. In Fig. 4.4, a situation in which a laparotomy was performed with the intention to resect the left liver lobe is shown. Intraoperatively, the cirrhosis appeared to be more advanced than preoperatively expected, and the amount of liver parenchyma that would have been resected appeared to be too large. We decided to perform a RFA instead as shown. Using the intraoperative ultrasound, a perfect placement of the RFA electrode can be easily achieved, which is crucial for a successful ablation. The ablation process is then performed according to the company's protocol. The patient of Fig. 4.4 had a HCC with a diameter of 3 cm and received an ablation of 5 cm. A situation in which additional tumor nodules were found intraoperatively can also lead to an inoperable status. This is of significance in cirrhotic livers, but also in metastatic disease without underlying liver disease. The decision to perform a liver resection or a RFA has to be made intraoperatively by an experienced liver surgeon.

The open surgical approach can also be combined with liver resection. This procedure is recommended when bilobar tumors are present, but a resection of both sides would lead to a loss of too much liver parenchyma. The combination leads to an extension of the indication for liver resection (Pawlik et al. 2003; Tepel et al. 2004). We normally perform first the liver resection, which may be extended. When this larger part

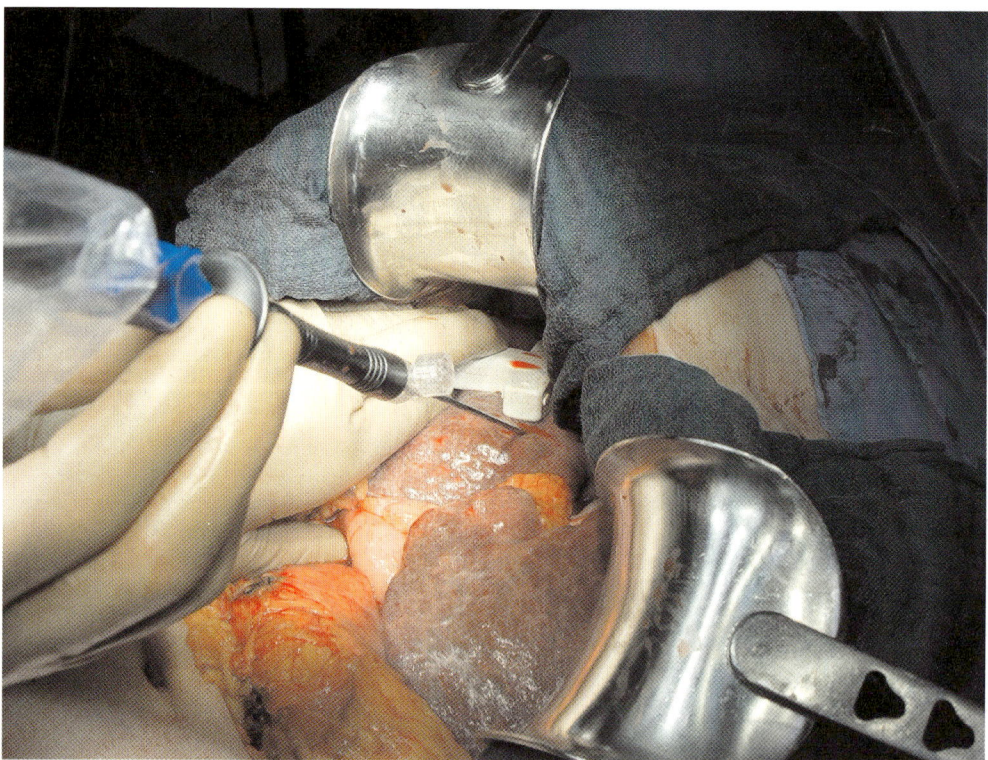

Fig. 4.4 RFA during open surgery in a cirrhotic liver. The HCC is located in segment IV. It was decided intraoperatively to perform RFA instead of resection

of the surgical therapy was successful without intraoperative complications, we perform the RFA as the smaller part of the therapy according to the previously described procedure during the same operation. Examples of this combined approach are a right hemihepatectomy combined with RFA deeply in segment IV, or a resection of the left lateral segments (II and III) combined with a RFA for tumors in the right liver lobe. Figure 4.5 illustrates CT scans of a combination of right hemihepatectomy and RFA in the left liver lobe. For liver resections, we perform a complete transverse laparotomy with median extension to the xiphoid process, or only an epigastric midline incision with extension as a right transverse incision (L-shaped incision). The liver is usually mobilized either on the right or the left side, depending on the location of the tumors.

4.4.4 Combination of the Laparoscopic and the Open Surgical Technique (Hand-Assisted Laparoscopic Radiofrequency Ablation)

This approach is not performed routinely by most centers, but may be used for particular indications. The advantages of the laparoscopic approach cannot always be realized for different reasons. It enables us to combine most of the advantages of the laparoscopic RFA with the advantages of the open surgical approach. The procedure is well tolerated by patients, as seen in our own experience with seven patients. All patients received a laparotomy of 8–10 cm in the epigastrium or hypogastrium, then severe adhesions were removed in three patients who had had previous surgery. After insertion of the hand-port, a periumbilical incision was made

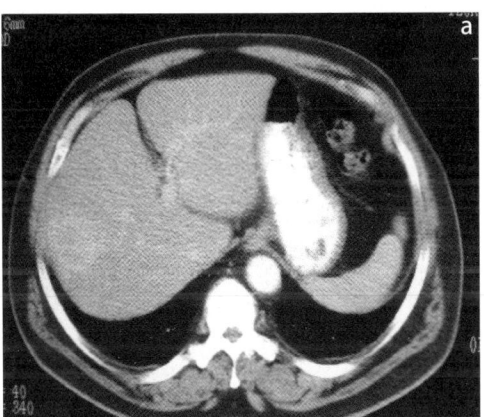
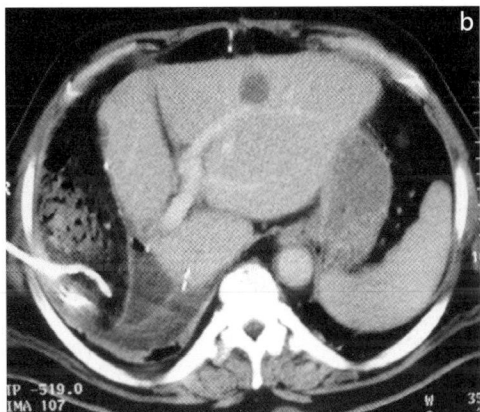
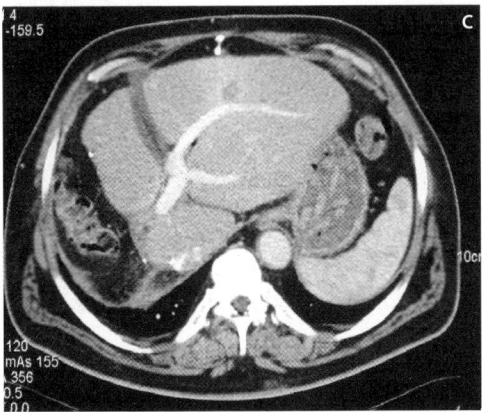

Fig. 4.5a–c CT scans of a liver with a colorectal liver metastasis in the right liver lobe. During right hemihepatectomy, an additional tumor in the left lateral segments was detected by intraoperative ultrasound, which was ablated with RFA during the same operation. **a** Preoperative situation. Only the tumor in right liver lobe was diagnosed preoperatively. **b** Follow-up 2 weeks after resection and RFA. **c** Follow-up 4 months after resection and RFA. Liver regeneration has occurred. The ablation site is still visible as a cyst after 4 months

and the camera was inserted safely. After insufflation of CO2 gas to reach an intra-abdominal pressure of 15 mm Hg, a complete laparoscopy was performed to reveal a possible peritoneal carcinomatosis. A thorough ultrasound examination of the whole liver was then preformed using a conventional open intraoperative ultrasound probe, and the tumors were localized. To achieve the easiest access to the tumors, another 5-mm trocar was inserted on the right side of the abdominal wall. The access to the abdominal wall consisted of the hand-port, the camera, a 5-mm trocar, and the RFA electrode. A monopolar electrode was inserted to perform adhesiolysis (Fig. 4.6a) and to mobilize the right liver lobe according to the location of the tumors (Fig. 4.6b). In case of tumors in segment VI (n = 4), the right liver lobe was mobilized nearly completely. During that maneuver, the liver was held back with the surgeon's right hand. A surgical towel was placed under the right liver lobe to protect adjacent organs such as the colon, diaphragm, kidney, and adrenal gland. This maneuver enables the most accurate ultrasound and placement of the electrode. The RFA electrode was inserted percutaneously and placed in the tumor under ultrasound guidance. The ablation process was initiated according to the company's protocol using the RITA Medical device. The recovery period for these patients is slightly longer than after laparoscopy with a discharge from the hospital 3 days after RFA. Machi et al. have reported similar results (Machi et al. 2002). It is an approach for RFA which has to be chosen individually by the surgeon and the patient.

4.5 Complications After Radiofrequency Ablation

The complication rate after RFA has been reported to be 8.9% in an exhaustive review of the world literature covering approximately 3,670 patients (Mulier et al. 2002). According to this meta-analysis, the complication rate observed after percutaneous RFA was 7.2%. The complication rate increased with the extent of the intervention with 9.5%, 9.9%, and 31.8% after a laparoscopic, simple open, and combined open approaches, respectively. The complications consisted of abdominal bleeding in 1.6%, abdominal infection in 1.1%, biliary tract damage in 1.0%, liver failure in 0.8%, pulmonary complications in 0.8%, dispersive pad skin burn in 0.6%, hepatic vascular damage in 0.6%, visceral damage in 0.5%, cardiac complications in 0.4%, myoglobinemia or myoglobinuria in 0.2%, renal failure in 0.1%, tumor seeding in 0.2%, coagulopathy in 0.2%, and hormonal complications in 0.1%. Another single-center series reported a total complication rate of 20.3% after RFA, including combinations of RFA and liver resection. RFA-related complications were seen in up to 9.8% (Jansen et al. 2005; Zagoria et al. 2002). In this series, the complications consisted of 19 major complications related to ten procedures. Two patients died from complications related to liver resection (1.4%). Other complications were observed with biliary tract damage (5.7%), liver failure (3.3%), hepatic abscess (2.5%), peritoneal infection (1.6%), intrahepatic hematoma (0.8%), hepatic artery aneurysm (0.8%), and pulmonary embolism (0.8%).

With adequate knowledge, many complications could be preventable. It is important to estimate the preoperative risk. The approach, whether it be percutaneous, laparoscopic, or surgical, has to be chosen according the location of the tumor. It is well known that the percutaneous approach should be avoided when the tumor is located on the liver surface. Liver function must be assessed preoperatively. Patients with Child C cirrhosis present with small livers and ascites. Portal hypertension, low platelet counts, and decreased clotting factors favor bleeding and liver failure, when the ablation zone becomes relatively large for a small liver with impaired function. When infections are known, such as sepsis, the ablation zone will be an ideal nidus for infection with the development of an abscess. After

Fig. 4.6 Hand-assisted laparoscopy. The right hand is inserted and used to retract tissue. a Adhesiolysis after previous surgery. b Mobilization of the right liver lobe. The hand raises the right liver lobe during mobilization using electrocautery

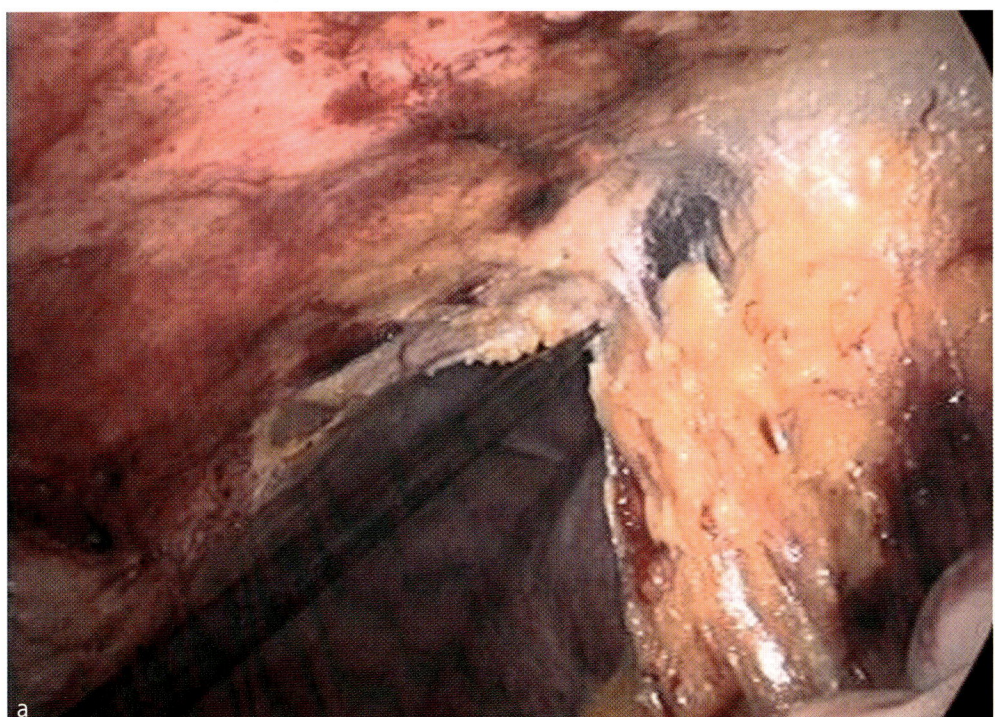

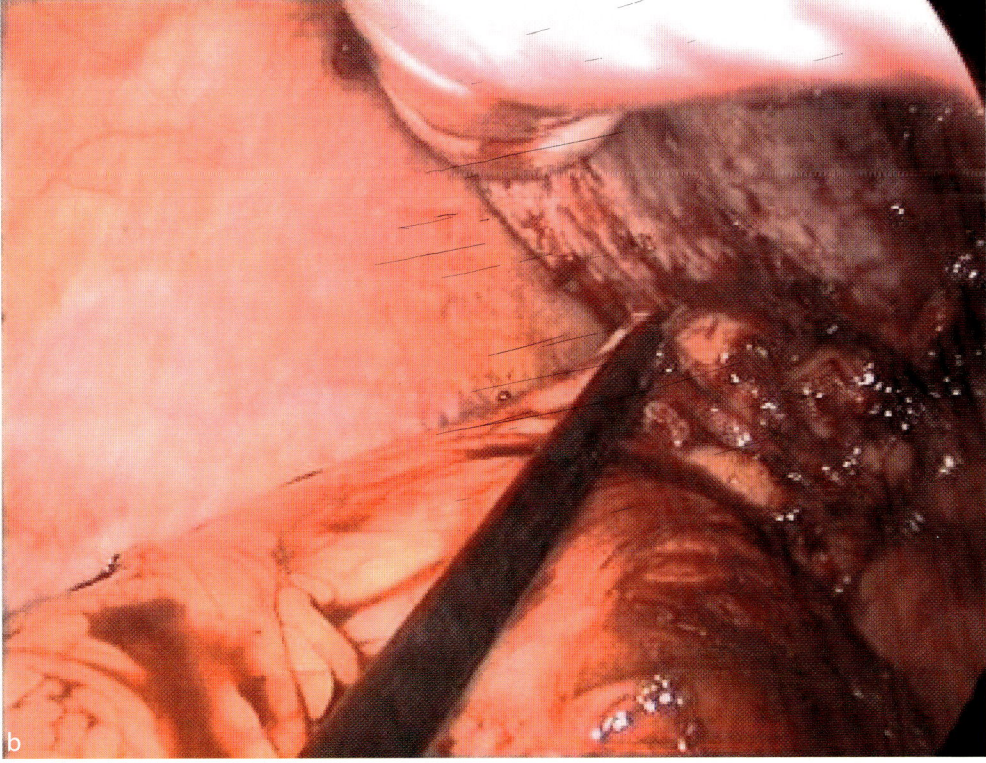

biliodigestive anastomosis, ascending cholangitis will also favor the development of abscesses in the ablation zone, which is therefore considered to be a contraindication for RFA.

The complications may be distinguished in RFA ablation-specific and approach-specific complications. In the following section, we will discuss the approaches to specific complications after laparoscopic and open surgical RFA.

4.5.1 Ablation-Specific Complications

RFA ablation-specific complications include damage by heat and coagulation, which may occur during percutaneous, laparoscopic, or open surgical RFA. Complications caused by heat from the RFA electrode include perforation of organs such as the stomach, duodenum, or colon. Less frequent is damage to the diaphragm or the bile ducts. The perforation of the stomach, duodenum, and colon can be avoided, when the RFA is laparoscopic or open surgery. Thermal injury of bile ducts can also be less frequent when a surgical approach for RFA is used because of the more precise placement of the electrode. The most frequent complication that is independent of the approach is the formation of abscesses. In a large study on 312 patients who underwent 350 sessions of radiofrequency ablation for treatment of 582 liver tumors, seven patients suffered from postinterventional formation of abscesses. Abscesses were seen more frequently in patients who had a bilioenteric anastomosis (3/3) than in other patients (4/223) ($p < 0.00001$) (de Baere et al. 2003). This increased abscess formation in the presence of bilioenteric anastomosis is caused by ascending bile duct infection.

4.5.2 Approach-Specific Complications

Approach-specific complications are mostly seen during the percutaneous approach, because organs in proximity to the liver cannot be protected as they can during surgical RFA. Another rare complication during percutaneous RFA is the development of pneumothorax because of the lack of direct visualization.

Complications during and after laparoscopic RFA are mainly caused by the laparoscopy itself. This includes injury of vessels or organs with cannulas or trocars, especially in previously operated patients with intra-abdominal adhesions.

Complications from the open surgical approach are, like the laparoscopic approach, not caused by the RFA but by the laparotomy itself. Most complications observed after this approach are caused by liver failure or complications due to a combined liver resection.

4.6 Summary

Radiofrequency ablation for the treatment of liver tumors is one of the best alternative treatment modalities when surgical resection is not possible. To find the right indication for the treatment, every patient should be treated in a high-volume center for the treatment of liver tumors in an interdisciplinary conference consisting of liver surgeons, interventional radiologists, medical oncologists, and gastroenterologists. With a multimodal approach including anatomic segmental and wedge resection of the liver, RFA, and chemotherapy, a median survival of 36 months was achieved in technically unresectable patients with colorectal liver metastases (Elias et al. 2005). This survival doubles the survival rate of any other treatment modality in this group of patients. These interdisciplinary conferences also serve to determine the approach for RFA, whether it should be percutaneous, laparoscopic, or open surgery. The safest ablation with the fewest adverse events from RFA is the open surgical approach, followed by the laparoscopic approach. The approach with the highest risk of injury to organs in proximity to the liver is the percutaneous approach. Therefore, many variables must be evaluated before making definite decisions.

After choosing RFA as the best alternative treatment option after evaluation of all variables for a particular patient, it offers a treatment option with a potential cure. A major advantage is the possible combination with liver resection, which extends the indication for surgical or ablative therapy.

References

1. Bentrem DJ, Dematteo RP, Blumgart LH (2005) Surgical therapy for metastatic disease to the liver. Annu Rev Med 56:139–156
2. De Baere T, Risse O, Kuoch V, Dromain C, Sengel C, Smayra T, Gamal El Din M, Letoublon C, Elias D (2003) Adverse events during radiofrequency treatment of 582 hepatic tumors. AJR Am J Roentgenol 181:695–700
3. Elias D, Baton O, Sideris L, Boige V, Malka D, Liberale G, Pocard M, Lasser P (2005) Hepatectomy plus intraoperative radiofrequency ablation and chemotherapy to treat technically unresectable multiple colorectal liver metastases. J Surg Oncol 90:36–42
4. Fong Y, Cohen AM, Fortner JG, Enker WE, Turnbull AD, Coit DG, Marrero AM, Prasad M, Blumgart LH, Brennan MF (1997) Liver resection for colorectal metastases. J Clin Oncol 15:938–946
5. Hoffman AL, Wu SS, Obaid AK, French SW, Lois J, McMonigle M, Ramos HC, Sher LS, Lopez RR (2002) Histologic evaluation and treatment outcome after sequential radiofrequency ablation and hepatic resection for primary and metastatic tumors. Am Surg 68:1038–1043
6. Jansen MC, van Duijnhoven FH, van Hillegersberg R, Rijken A, van Coevorden F, van der Sijp J, Prevoo W, van Gulik TM (2005) Adverse effects of radiofrequency ablation of liver tumours in the Netherlands. Br J Surg 92:1248–1254
7. Jonas S, Bechstein WO, Steinmuller T, Herrmann M, Radke C, Berg T, Settmacher U, Neuhaus P (2001) Vascular invasion and histopathologic grading determine outcome after liver transplantation for hepatocellular carcinoma in cirrhosis. Hepatology 33:1080–1086
8. Kapoor BS, Hunter DW (2003) Injection of subphrenic saline during radiofrequency ablation to minimize diaphragmatic injury. Cardiovasc Intervent Radiol 26:302–304
9. Kokudo N, Bandai Y, Imanishi H, Minagawa M, Uedera Y, Harihara Y, Makuuchi M (1996) Management of new hepatic nodules detected by intraoperative ultrasonography during hepatic resection for hepatocellular carcinoma. Surgery 119:634–640
10. Leonard GD, Brenner B, Kemeny NE (2005) Neoadjuvant chemotherapy before liver resection for patients with unresectable liver metastases from colorectal carcinoma. J Clin Oncol 23:2038–2048
11. Machi J, Oishi AJ, Mossing AJ, Furumoto NL, Oishi RH (2002) Hand-assisted laparoscopic ultrasound-guided radiofrequency thermal ablation of liver tumors: a technical report. Surg Laparosc Endosc Percutan Tech 12:160–164
12. Montorsi M, Santambrogio R, Bianchi P, Opocher E, Zuin M, Bertolini E, Bruno S, Podda M (2001) Radiofrequency interstitial thermal ablation of hepatocellular carcinoma in liver cirrhosis. Role of the laparoscopic approach. Surg Endosc 15:141–145
13. Mulier S, Mulier P, Ni Y, Miao Y, Dupas B, Marchal G, De Wever I, Michel L (2002) Complications of radiofrequency coagulation of liver tumours. Br J Surg 89:1206–1222
14. Pascher A, Jonas S, Neuhaus P (2003) Intrahepatic cholangiocarcinoma: indication for transplantation. J Hepatobiliary Pancreat Surg 10:282–287
15. Pawlik TM, Izzo F, Cohen DS, Morris JS, Curley SA (2003) Combined resection and radiofrequency ablation for advanced hepatic malignancies: results in 172 patients. Ann Surg Oncol 10:1059–1069
16. Scheele J, Stang R, Altendorf-Hofmann A, Paul M (1995) Resection of colorectal liver metastases. World J Surg 19:59–71
17. Scott DJ, Young WN, Watumull LM, Lindberg G, Fleming JB, Huth JF, Rege RV, Jeyarajah DR, Jones DB (2001) Accuracy and effectiveness of laparoscopic vs open hepatic radiofrequency ablation. Surg Endosc 15:135–140
18. Scott DJ, Fleming JB, Watumull LM, Lindberg G, Tesfay ST, Jones DB (2002) The effect of hepatic inflow occlusion on laparoscopic radiofrequency ablation using simulated tumors. Surg Endosc 16:1286–1291
19. Shen P, Fleming S, Westcott C, Challa V (2003) Laparoscopic radiofrequency ablation of the liver in proximity to major vasculature: effect of the Pringle maneuver. J Surg Oncol 83:36–41

20. Siperstein A, Garland A, Engle K, Rogers S, Berber E, Foroutani A, String A, Ryan T, Ituarte P (2000) Local recurrence after laparoscopic radiofrequency thermal ablation of hepatic tumors. Ann Surg Oncol 7:106–113
21. Smith MK, Mutter D, Forbes LE, Mulier S, Marescaux J (2004) The physiologic effect of the pneumoperitoneum on radiofrequency ablation. Surg Endosc 18:35–38
22. Tepel J, Hinz S, Klomp HJ, Kapischke M, Kremer B (2004) Intraoperative radiofrequency ablation (RFA) for irresectable liver malignancies. Eur J Surg Oncol 30:551–555
23. Wiersinga WJ, Jansen MC, Straatsburg IH, Davids PH, Klaase JM, Gouma DJ, van Gulik TM (2003) Lesion progression with time and the effect of vascular occlusion following radiofrequency ablation of the liver. Br J Surg 90:306–312
24. Zagoria RJ, Chen MY, Shen P, Levine EA (2002) Complications from radiofrequency ablation of liver metastases. Am Surg 68:204–209

5 Laser-Induced Thermotherapy

Birger Mensel, Christiane Weigel, Norbert Hosten

Recent Results in Cancer Research, Vol. 167
© Springer-Verlag Berlin Heidelberg 2006

5.1 Introduction

Laser-induced interstitial thermotherapy is a method for controlled tissue destruction. Cells compounds are destroyed in situ by hyperthermia. Laser-induced thermotherapy (LITT) is able to induce a circumscript necrosis in targeted tissue while maximally surrounding tissue. The first patients were treated 20 years ago and possible gains in therapy of oncologic patients were quickly recognized. LITT has gained broad clinical acceptance in numerous centers during the last 10 years. Advantages of LITT in the treatment of cancer patients are the minimally invasive nature of LITT with percutaneous tissue access under image guidance; the limited investment in hardware and the limited time necessary for a treatment; the possibility of treating patients in analgo-sedation, thus minimizing hospitalization; and the possibility of treating patients after other therapeutic options have failed. The database today is broadest for liver tumors; metastases, foremost of colorectal carcinoma and hepatocellular carcinoma, are tumors treated in large numbers. Lesions in other locations, however, are treated in growing numbers, among them lung tumors, advanced head and neck tumors, renal cell carcinoma, and osteoid osteomas. There is also experience in treatment of brain tumors, prostatic cancer, and pancreatic carcinoma, the latter being of an experimental nature. Modification of the applicators for special indications has broadened the therapeutic spectrum of LITT. LITT is uniquely suited for monitoring by imaging, namely MRI. CT and ultrasound may also be used for some types of thermoimaging, with each of these methods having specific advantages and disadvantages.

5.2 Technical Aspects of Laser-Induced Thermotherapy

The principle of LITT is introduction of laser radiation into tissue while the laser is in contact with tissue. Interaction between laser radiation and tissue results in transformation of laser radiation into thermic energy, which induces three-dimensional coagulation necrosis if the temperature is successfully kept at a thermotoxic level for a sufficiently long time. The diameter of the resulting necrosis depends on the characteristics of the laser used and of the heated tissue.

5.2.1 Physics of Laser Radiation

Laser is an acronym for light amplification of stimulated emission of radiation. Radiation emitted from a laser generator is electromagnetic waves, which are coherent, collimated, and monochromatic. Laser waves are generated in a laser medium by charging processes in the atomic dimension. The charging may be optical, chemical, or electrical. Laser light is generated when charged electrons fall from a higher to a lower level of energy. Energy released during this process is released as light. This process of induced emission results in laser enhancement: a first photon induces the decay of a second photon of identical phase and wavelength. When certain laser media are being used, laser radiation suited for medical use may result. For LITT, the neodymium:yttrium-aluminium-garnet (Nd:YAG) laser is especially suited. It has a wavelength of 1064 nm, in the near infrared part of the spectrum. The Nd:YAG laser easily transmits energy and is characterized by a high optical penetration into tissue (Roggan et al. 1995).

5.2.2 Interaction Between Laser Radiation and Biological Tissue

At the interface of laser radiation and biological tissue, photons of laser radiation interact with atoms of tissue. Different effects result. Laser light is distributed spatially in the volume it enters. Laser sources with wavelengths in the near infrared part of the spectrum, as they are used in LITT, penetrate deeply into tissue. Optical penetration is on the order of 2–10 mm. Three processes characterize distribution of laser light in target tissue and the resulting effects: absorption, scattering, and bending. Biological effects of laser light are ultimately based on the transformation of laser energy into thermal energy. Photons are absorbed on an atomic and molecular level in different depths of the tissue thus irradiated by laser light. Depending on the thermic capacity of the tissue, a different temperature results. For laser radiation with a wavelength in the near infrared part of the spectrum, absorption is mainly determined by water and hemoglobin content. More generally, the degree of absorption is influenced by laser wavelength and the optical characteristics of tissue. These are described by the absorption coefficient (μ_a), scattering coefficient (μ_s), and the anisotropy factor (g, another parameter describing scattering). On deeper layers of tissue, the proportion of radiation being absorbed decreases (the Lambert Beer law). The amount of thermal energy deposited per volume and ultimately the resulting temperature decreases. During LITT, optical, thermal, and mechanical tissue characteristics change due to heating. Distribution of laser light in these tissues and the gradient of the resulting temperature change (Beuthan et al. 1992; Roggan et al. 1995).

5.2.2.1 Thermal Effects and Tissue Effects

LITT results in heating the tissue volume under treatment. The aim of LITT is complete destruction of malignant tissues. The basic concept of LITT is that of classical hyperthermia, which postulates an increased sensitivity of malignant cells to exposure to heat due to its hypoxic metabolism (Bhuyan 1979). It should be noted, however, that LITT works in a higher temperature range than hyperthermia (60–100 °C). The hyperthermic effect is thus complemented by tissue coagulation. The increase in temperature, which is actually observed, depends not on optical characteristics alone but also on tissue characteristics such as heat capacity and heat convectability).

Thermally induced tissue necroses result from temperature increases beyond 43 °C with the time until cell death depending exponentially on temperature. Locally increased temperature induces a variety of processes, among them induction of enzymes, denaturation of proteins and collagen, and sclerosing of vessels. These phenomena can result in cell death alone or in sum. A carbonization of tissue, however, should be avoided, as it changes optical characteristics of tissue in such a way that laser light is for the most part absorbed, penetration of photons is limited, and the volume of coagulation that can be finally achieved is restricted.

5.2.3 Laser Fibers and Laser Applicators

Transmission of laser energy is achieved by laser fibers (optical fibers). They transmit the visible light and light of the near infrared part of the spectrum with practically no loss and over large distances. Quartz fibers have proven to be well suited for transmission of laser light during LITT. Laser fibers may be destroyed when they absorb part of the laser energy. Quartz fibers are characterized by minimal losses due to absorption for light with a wavelength between 200 and 2000 nm. They are heat-resistant and flexible. They enable near lossless transmission of the high-power density of the laser ray between the laser generator and the laser applicator (Schönborn 1993). The tip of the laser fibers, which has contact with the tissue under therapy, is modified according to the LITT specification. Applicators of different designs exist, among them ring-mode, bare fibers, and zebra applicators. Cooled diffuser tip applicators have, however, proved most practical for LITT. They are characterized by spherical emission of energy and produce well-defined 3D coagulation necrosis (Steeger et al. 1992; Roggan et al. 1995). Cooled laser applicators differ in their diameter. If the cooling medium is moved in a closed circuit, they have a large diameter because of the need for an inlet and an outlet for the cooling medium, which cools the diffuser tip. If the applicator is open at the tip and the cooling medium allowes vaporizing the diameter is smaller (Hosten et al. 2003; Puls et al. 2003). In the latter design, the cooling medium is pumped through the thin space between the applicator and the laser fiber. Cooling medium vaporizes at the distal orifice of the applicator and ultimately condenses in tissue. Because the space between the laser fiber and the applicator is small, the flow necessary to avoid carbonization may be kept extremely low (0.75 ml/min). The amount of cooling medium needed for a treatment session is thus very small, making recycling unnecessary. The diameter of open-tip applicators is therefore small. Compared to 9F inlet/outlet applicators, the diameter of open-tip applicators may be reduced by 40% to 5.5F (Fig. 5.1). The system may be positioned directly in tissue compared to the Seldinger technique commonly used for applicators with larger diameters. For positioning, a titanium mandrin is introduced into the Teflon applicator, which is replaced by the laser fiber after the applicator is in position. The miniaturized applicator combines the advantages of large diameter, cooled applicators with the smaller diameter of an uncooled applicator. Minimal invasiveness is thus combined with optimized efficacy of laser transmission. Tumors in organs such as the lungs, where invasiveness must be kept to a minimum can thus be treated.

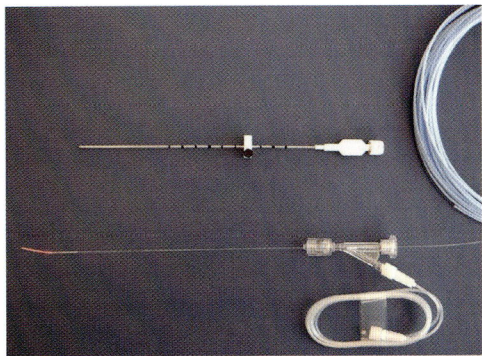

Fig. 5.1 Miniaturized applicator with open tip. The *upper part* shows the applicator with Teflon tubing and the inserted mandrin. After placement of the applicator, the mandrin is exchanged for the laser fiber (*lower part*). The y-shaped distributor connects the Teflon tube to the line that transports the cooling medium

5.2.4 Imaging Temperature Distribution

LITT has the unique advantage of allowing on-line MR thermometry. GRE sequences show signal loss in regions where temperature is increased. There is a correlation between temperature and signal reduction, though whether this reflects temperature or a secondary phenomenon is not clear. Parameter images showing actual isotherms may be generated from MR examinations. This has the advantage that ablation times can be individually chosen, i.e., laser energy is introduced into a metastasis until on-line thermometry demonstrates that the 90 °C isotherm covers the metastasis plus a safety margin of 1 cm. As other ablation therapies do not allow ablation while on-line MR thermometry is performed (radiofrequency ablation) or do not generate phenomena that can be imaged (brachytherapy), other imaging modalities were tried. Ultrasound and CT actually demonstrate some changes in imaging during radiofrequency but whether this is directly temperature-related or corresponds to gas formation is not yet clear.

5.2.5 Application

Laser-induced thermotherapy can be optimized in different ways:

Single-applicator technique. This technique percutaneously places a single applicator; it is removed when therapy is completed. If very large tumors need to be treated, two approaches are possible.

Multiple applicator technique using multiple entries. Between two and five applicators are placed inside one tumor. Heat application is simultaneous. Distances between applicators must be optimized in such a way that applicators are neither burned by neighboring applicators, nor are there low-temperature areas resulting in an insufficient tumoricidal effect. Ideally, a homogeneous ablation zone results, which is larger than that achieved by five single ablations.

Multiple applicator technique using a single entry. For this technique, a single applicator is used for multiple ablations by pulling is back inside the needle tract once ablation at a certain point is achieved. Ideally, a large, oval ablation volume results. Multiple applicators may additionally be pulled back simultaneously (Vogl et al. 2000).

5.3 Laser-Induced Thermotherapy of Liver Tumors

While multiple organs are within the reach of LITT, clinical experience is greatest for metastases to the liver and lungs. Brain tumors have been treated for some time by LITT, while bone metastases and benign bone lesions are more recent targets of clinical research.

5.4 Clinical Results – Laser-Induced Thermotherapy of Liver Metastases

Therapy of primary or secondary liver tumors is a frequent problem in clinical routine. With liver metastases accounting for 90% of all malignant liver lesions, they constitute the biggest challenge. The large number of liver metastases is the result of the liver's role as central organ of Stoffwechsel: it is a filter between the portal and the caval vessel system and therefore prevents malignant cells entering the general circulation. For many tumor entities, liver metastasis is the limiting factor for survival. This holds true especially for gastrointestinal tumors where the liver is the first and often the sole target of hematogenous metastases. Of all patients with colorectal cancer, 25% have liver metastases at the time of diagnosis; 50% develop liver metastases with time. Efficacy of surgical therapy is limited because only 30% of all patients with liver metastases from colorectal primaries can be operated; in more than 50% of all patients with R0 resection, liver metastases recur (Jaeck et al. 1997). All these facts make thermoablative therapies such as LITT so important clinically.

Inclusion criteria for treatment by LITT are a number of lesions not exceeding five (analogous to criteria for surgical resection); no lesion has a diameter of more than 5 cm (technical limit); absence of extrahepatic metastases; relapsing metastasis after surgical resection; metastasis to both lobes of the liver (LITT in combination with surgical removal); and patients whose clinical state does not allow for surgery or who do not consent. Several studies describe results of LITT of liver metastases and hepatocellular carcinoma. Vogl et al. treated 603 patients with 1801 liver metastases in 1555 sessions. They placed the applicators under CT guidance and monitored temperature during ablation by MRI. Local progress after 6 months was observed in 4.4% of patients with tumors measuring more than 4.0 cm, 1.2% for lesions larger between 3.1 and 4.0 cm, 2.4% between 21. and 3.0 cm, and 1.9% for lesions less than 2.0 cm in diameter. Mean survival after diagnosis was 4.4 years (median, 3.5 years) for all patients with 1-, 2- to 3-, and 5-year survival rates of 90%, 77%, 56%, and 37%, respectively. One patient died within 30 days after intervention. Major complications were pleural effusion (17 cases), intra-abdominal bleeding (two patients), liver abscess (n = 6) and one case of pneumothorax, a lesion of the biliary tract, and bronchobiliary fistula each. The study

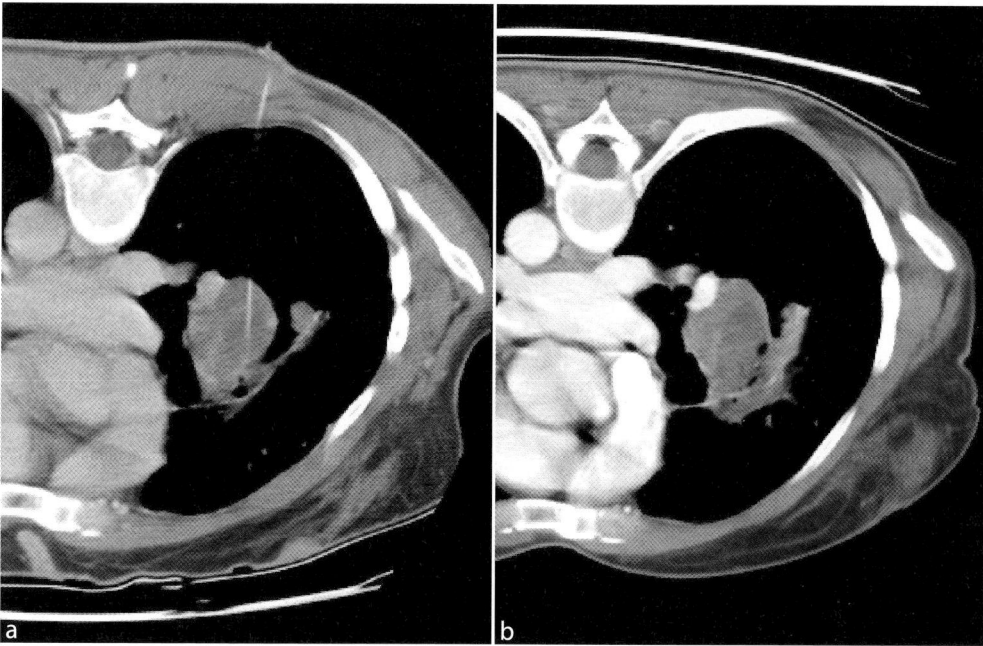

Fig. 5.2 Effect of laser ablation on lung metastases. The *left part* of the image was obtained during LITT with the applicator and the laser fiber in situ. The *right part* was obtained 3 weeks later after infusion of contrast medium. Note that there is an area of reduced perfusion surrounding the laser fiber corresponding to the area, which may be ablated with one applicator in one session. For complete coverage of a lesion of the size shown, multiple applicators can be positioned or a single applicator can be repositioned or treatment can be repeated. The latter option was chosen in this case

also demonstrated that small tumors may be more effectively treated than larger ones; patients treated with cooled applicators preventing carbonization had significantly better survival than those treated with uncooled applicators (Vogl et al. 2004). For 39 patients with hepatocellular carcinoma treated by LITT, Eichler et al. found a technical efficacy of 97.5%. Applicator placement was CT-guided and therapy was performed under MRI monitoring. No major complications were observed (Eichler et al. 2001). A recent paper by our group showed that LITT may safely and effectively treat lesions located close to large vessels in the liver hilum (Mensel et al. 2005). Survival was comparable to that observed after LITT of peripheral liver metastases.

Study design is mainly flawed in patient selection. Prospective, controlled studies could never be performed due to patient preferences. Published studies necessarily include patients treated with a variety of chemotherapies both before and after LITT.

In conclusion, LITT has a technical efficacy greater than 90%. Mortality is less than 0.1%. Mean survival is more than 4 years when patients are selected according to accepted inclusion and exclusion criteria. Frequent complications are pleural effusion and intrahepatic or subcapsular hematoma (Mack et al. 2004; Vogl et al. 2004). Survival rates for LITT are comparable to those after R0 resection, but both mortality and complications are significantly lower. Indications for LITT of liver lesions are more than for operation.

5.5 Clinical Results – Laser-Induced Thermotherapy of Lung Metastases

Our group has performed lung tumour ablation with a thin-caliber laser applicator system with open tip since 2001. Forty-two patients with 64 lung tumors were treated (39 patients with metastases and three with primary tumors). Fourteen lesions were central and 50 were peripheral. Mean follow-up was 7.6 months (range, 6 weeks to 39 months). Eighty percent of treatments were technically successful in the first session. Pneumothorax was the main complication and occurred in 50% of the first 20 patients and in 35% of the rest. Two patients required a chest tube. It took several weeks for the effect of therapy to become apparent on follow-up CT (Fig. 5.2). Thirty-nine percent of all lesions increased in size immediately after treatment. Gross reduction in size with scar formation was seen in 50% of the lesions and cavitations in 13%. Local tumor control was achieved in 51 lesions; 9% of lesions that were less than 1.5 cm progressed despite therapy and progress was observed in more than 11% of larger lesions. Progression was also more frequent in lesions located in the basal parts of the lung (47%).

5.6 Outlook

LITT with an open-tip applicator is suited for the treatment of liver and lung tumors. In lung metastases, lesions located centrally and in the upper parts of the lungs are more easily accessible to treatment than lesions located peripherally and close to the diaphragm. Lesions of medium size show better results than either very small (< 1 cm) or very large lesions (> 5 cm). The open-tip applicator has the potential for infusion of tumoricide substances.

References

1. Beuthan J, Gewiese B, Wolf KJ, Müller G (1992) Die laserinduzierte Thermotherapie (LITT)-biophysikalische Aspekte ihrer Anwendung. Med Tech 3:102–106
2. Bhuyan BK (1979) Kinetics of cell kill by hyperthermia. Cancer Res 39:2277–2284
3. Eichler K, Mack MG, Straub R, Engelmann K, Zangos S, Woitaschek D, Vogl TJ (2001) [Oligonodular hepatocellular carcinoma (HCC): MR-controlled laser-induced thermotherapy]. Radiologe 41:915–922
4. Hosten N, Stier A, Weigel C, Kirsch M, Puls R, Nerger U, Jahn D, Stroszczynski C, Heidecke CD, Speck U (2003) [Laser-induced thermotherapy (LITT) of lung metastases: description of a miniaturized applicator, optimization, and initial treatment of patients]. Rofo 175:393–400
5. Jaeck D, Bachellier P, Guiguet M, Boudjema K, Vaillant JC, Balladur P, Nordlinger B (1997) Long-term survival following resection of colorectal hepatic metastases. Association Française de Chirurgie. Br J Surg 84:977–980
6. Mack MG, Straub R, Eichler K, Sollner O, Lehnert T, Vogl TJ (2004) Breast cancer metastases in liver: laser-induced interstitial thermotherapy – local tumor control rate and survival data. Radiology 233:400–409
7. Mensel B, Weigel C, Heidecke CD, Stier A, Hosten N (2005) [Laser-induced thermotherapy (LITT) of tumors of the liver in central location: results and complications]. Rofo 177:1267–1275
8. Puls R, Stroszczynski C, Gaffke G, Hosten N, Felix R, Speck U (2003) Laser-induced thermotherapy (LITT) of liver metastases: MR-guided percutaneous insertion of an MRI-compatible irrigated microcatheter system using a closed high-field unit. J Magn Reson Imaging 17:663–670
9. Roggan A, Albrecht D, Berlien H-P, Beuthan J, Fuchs B (1995) Application equipment for intraoperative and percutaneous laser-induced interstitial thermotherapy (LITT). In: Müller G, Roggan A (eds) Laser-induced thermotherapy. Spie Optical Engineering Press, Bellingham, pp 224–248

10. Roggan A, Dörschel K, Minet O, Wolff D, Müller G (1995) The optical properties of biological tissue in the near infrared wavelength range – review and measurements. In: Müller G, Roggan A (eds) Laser-induced thermotherapy. Spie Optical Engineering Press, Bellingham, pp 10–44
11. Schönborn K-H (1993) Lichtwellenleiter. In: Berlien HP, Müller G (eds) Angewandte Lasermedizin Lehr-und Handbuch für Praxis und Klinik. ecomed Verlagsgesellschaft mbH, Landsberg-München, pp 1–10
12. Steger AC, Lees WR, Shorvon P, Walmsley K, Bown SG (1992) Multiple-fibre low-power interstitial laser hyperthermia: studies in the normal liver. Br J Surg 79:139–145
13. Vogl TJ, Mack M, Straub R, Eichler K, Engelmann K, Roggan A, Zangos S (2000) Perkutane interstitielle Thermotherapie maligner Lebertumore. Rofo 172:12 22
14. Vogl TJ, Straub R, Eichler K, Sollner O, Mack MG (2004) Colorectal carcinoma metastases in liver: laser-induced interstitial thermotherapy – local tumor control rate and survival data. Radiology 230:450–458

Part III Clinical Results of Minimally Invasive Tumor Therapies

6 Liver Metastases

Andreas Lubienski, Thorsten Leibecke, Karin Lubienski, Thomas Helmberger

6.1 Introduction

Image-guided minimally invasive treatment modalities for local tumor ablation in liver metastases have emerged during recent years not only as treatment alternatives in patients who cannot undergo resection, but as potential curative therapy in selected patients [1]. So far, several interstitial treatment modalities such as radiofrequency ablation (RFA), laser-induced thermotherapy (LITT), microwave ablation (PMCT), high-intensity focused ultrasound (HIFU), cryoablation, and percutaneous ethanol injection (PEI) have been introduced. Compared to other locally ablative techniques, RFA has gained the most widespread clinical and scientific acceptance documented by a significant number of articles during recent years.

Malignant tumors of the gastrointestinal tract represent the major cause for metastatic disease confined to the liver. Synchronous liver metastases occur in approximately 15%–25% of all patients, whereas 60%–80% will develop metachronous liver metastases after curative resection of the primary tumor during the course of the disease [2]. Surgical resection provides the greatest potential for cure in patients with secondary liver tumors but can be offered only to a small number of patients (5%–20%) [3]. In most centers, contraindications to resection include bilobar disease, more than six metastases, and unfavorable location of the tumors, endangering the functional integrity of the liver after resection. Survival rates range from 25% to 40% at 5 years [3, 4], with an operative mortality of about 2% in patients that undergo extended hepatic resection [5].

Morbidity ranges between 22% and 39%. The presence of lymph node involvement, extrahepatic metastases, advanced-stage, or poor differentiation of the primary is often associated with reduced survival. The characteristics of liver metastases associated with decreased survival included large size, increased number, satellite tumors, and bilobar distribution. Liver metastases that are discovered after a short disease-free interval after onset of the disease, synchronous metastases, and metastases associated with elevated CEA marker levels also predicted shorter survival [4]. Surgical resections with less than 1-cm tumor-free margin and extensive resections may be associated with decreased survival. In roughly 60%–75% of all resected patients (R0 resection), recurrent liver metastases will occur, with 85% of these detected within 2.5 years after diagnosis of the primary [6, 7]. Systemic chemotherapy is usually given as adjuvant or neoadjuvant treatment to hepatic resection and/or if resection is not possible. Dependent on the underlying tumor, median survival can reach 16–20 months with modern chemotherapy regimens in patients with colorectal liver metastases. Recent studies indicate that the additional application of monoclonal antibodies (e.g., Bevacizumab) can significantly prolong survival compared to the treatment with vascular endothelial growth factor [8]. However, in most cases long-term survival cannot be achieved with systemic chemotherapy and recurrent treatments with different regimens are necessary. Since there is no consensus on the role of local ablative treatments such as RFA in metastatic disease, the vast majority of patients with hepatic metastases are referred for RFA, usually in the late course of their disease after systemic chemotherapy. Nevertheless, even in this highly palliative situation, local tumor control by RFA is often equal or even better compared to systemic chemotherapy [9]. Therefore, it is of ample interest to implement local ablative therapies such as RFA in the treatment algorithm for nonresectable liver metastases.

6.2 Patient Selection

Patients with hepatic metastases who did not meet the selection criteria for hepatic surgery may be candidates for local ablative treatments based on the presence of liver-only disease [10, 11]. Since RFA is not yet a generally accepted first- or second-line treatment, it has to be considered as a palliative intention-to-treat therapy option. So far, no clear indications for the use of RFA in metastatic liver disease are defined. Therefore, the pros and cons have to be balanced optimally by an interdisciplinary team weighing potential partial benefits in terms of survival and/or quality of life vs potential risks and/or inefficacy (Table 6.1).

Given the limitations of currently available RF systems, RF treatment of tumors exceeding 4–5 cm in size should be avoided in order to minimize the risk of residual unablated tumor. Moderate to high rates of local tumor recurrence, especially of large tumors, have been reported [12, 13]. A possible reason for failures in the treatment of large tumors is the inability to determine the optimal number of ablations and the exact location of electrode placement needed to completely destroy tumors larger than the size of a single ablation zone To treat even larger tumors, multiple ablations need to be overlapped to build a composite thermal injury of sufficient size to kill the tumor and provide an adequate tumor-free margin [14, 15]. Dodd et al. [16] reported their results of computer analysis of the thermal injury sizes created by overlapping ablations and proposed six- and 14-ablation models. Their results demonstrated the importance of performing these types of calculations to develop tumor ablation strategies.

From a practical point of view, in most centers the number of hepatic tumors to be treated is limited to four or five. An on-going trial (chemotherapy + local ablation vs chemotherapy [CLOCC], sponsored by The European Organisation for Research and Treatment of Cancer [EORTC]) has more generous inclusion criteria. Patients can have as many as nine metastases with a maximum diameter of 4 cm [17]. Given the unique biology of metastatic neuroendocrine disease, surgical experience has shown that debulking of tumors can considerably improve patient survival and symptoms. However, there is no proven evidence of this concept in other tumor entities; one can even argue that aggressive ablation of hepatic metastases with destruction of more than 90% of the tumor burden could result in a benefit [18].

6.3 Follow-Up Imaging

Monitoring therapy effectiveness is deemed a major issue in interventional tumor therapy. Computed tomography (CT) and magnetic reso-

Table 6.1 Inclusion and exclusion criteria for RFA in liver metastases

Indications	Contraindications
No respectability	Untreatable systemic metastases
Work in progress: bilobar tumors prior to resection	Tumor load > 70% of the entire liver
< 4–5 Tumors	Coagulopathy
Tumor size < 4–5 cm	Septicemia
Resection refused by patient	Portal vein thrombosis

nance imaging (MRI) are, although widely used, of limited sensitivity, specificity, and accuracy when assessing the liver for residual tumor following RFA [19–21]. This limitation relates to their predominantly morphologic character, which can only partly be compensated by administration of contrast agents. The accuracy is limited by both spatial and contrast resolution to approximately 2–3 mm (depending on the imaging modality) [22]. Postprocedural imaging findings are only a rough guide to the success of ablation therapy, since microscopic foci of residual disease, by definition, cannot be expected to be identified. Despite these facts, dynamic contrast-enhanced CT and MRI are still playing a major role in follow-up imaging after RFA.

There are two types of imaging findings that can be identified after an ablation procedure: those related to zones of decreased or absent perfusion and those in which the signal intensity (at MR imaging) or attenuation (at CT) are altered [10, 23]. Because of the characteristics of some metastatic liver lesions (e.g., colorectal cancer) – relatively hypovascular compared to the normal liver tissue – interpretation of follow-up scans are sometimes difficult since contrast enhancement of viable tumor foci may not be present or only minor. In addition, a periablational enhancement may be seen in early follow-up scans. Especially in tumors that initially enhanced in contrast studies, rim enhancement after treatment might be confused with residual enhancing tumor tissue. Depending on the protocol used for contrast-enhanced imaging (injection rate and scanning delay), this transient finding can be seen immediately after ablation and can last for up to 6 months after ablation [24]. It usually manifests as a penumbra, or a thin rim peripheral to the zone of ablation, that can typically measure up to 5 mm (in the immediate postinterventional phase) but most often measures 1–2 mm. It is characterized by a relatively concentric, symmetric, and uniform enhancement with smooth inner margins that needs to be differentiated from irregular peripheral enhancement suspicious of recurrent or new tumor. The finding is most readily appreciated on the arterial phase CT scans, with persistent enhancement that is often seen on delayed MR images. Histopathologically, it represents a benign physiologic response to thermal injury (initially, reactive hyperemia; subsequently, fibrosis and giant cell reaction) [25]. In contrast, irregular peripheral enhancement represents residual tumor at the treatment margin often in a scattered, nodular, or eccentric pattern, indicating incomplete local treatment. Given the delayed enhancement characteristics of many hypovascular tumors, this finding is often best appreciated in a comparison of portal venous or delayed images (3 min or more after contrast material injection) with baseline images. Complete coagulation necrosis corresponds to a hypoattenuated area and fails to enhance after contrast injection. On MRI, the treated tumor is characterized by a low signal intensity on T2-weighted images, whereas viable tumor is shown to be hyperintense on T2-weighted images [26]. Biopsies of ablated areas in order to proof complete necrosis are generally unreliable and therefore not recommended [27]. The ablation of appropriate margins (0.5–1.0 cm) beyond the borders of the tumor is necessary to achieve complete tumor destruction [16]. Therefore, an ablation zone that is not larger than the tumor before ablation should be followed up closely. Long-term follow-up imaging may show a gradual decrease in the volume of the ablation zone considered to represent only residual necrotic or fibrotic tissue that is present during the absorption process [20]. It is important to note that no or minimal involution does not imply treatment failure. Many other imaging findings such as inflammatory stranding in the acute period after ablation and more chronic findings such as fibrosis, scarring, and architectural distortion that represent both host reaction to ablation and repair mechanisms will be seen.

When imaging and clinical findings at short-term follow-up are inconclusive and the suspected lesion is small, follow-up at 1- to 3-month intervals should be considered before performing an invasive diagnostic procedure such as percutaneous biopsy or retreatment [28]. In most centers, follow-up scans are performed in 3-month intervals and are often combined with serum tumor markers such as CEA [29, 30]. Any increase in lesion size or irregularity or residual enhancement should be carefully interpreted in terms of residual tumor foci or recurrent metastases (Fig. 6.1a,b). It is mandatory to look for

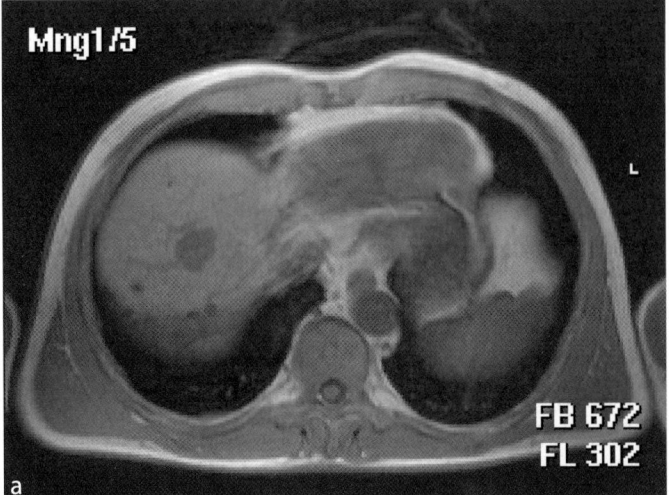

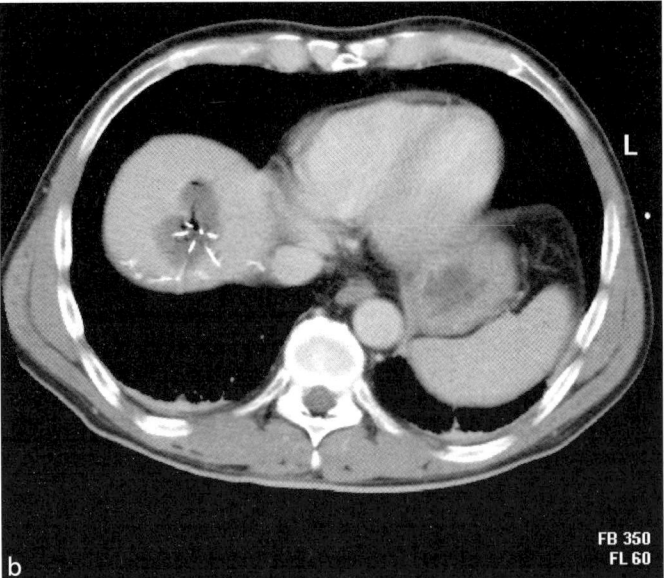

Fig. 6.1 a Nonenhanced MRI (T1 flash 2d; breath-hold; slice thickness, 8 mm) of a unifocal colorectal liver metastasis (diameter 3 cm) in the liver dome. b CT-guided RFA with the RF electrode (RITA, 3–5 cm; working length, 25 cm) in place. c Nonenhanced MRI (T1 flash 2d; breath hold; slice thickness, 8 mm) follow-up scan 1 month after RFA showing a hemorrhagic ablation zone (hyperintense area) encompassing the hypointense tumorous lesion with no evidence of residual tumor foci. d Nonenhanced MRI (T1 flash 2d; breath hold; slice thickness, 8 mm) follow-up scan 1 year after RFA showing the hemorrhagic ablation zone (hyperintense area) encompassing the hypointense tumorous lesion with no evidence of residual tumor foci. Note the tumor involution

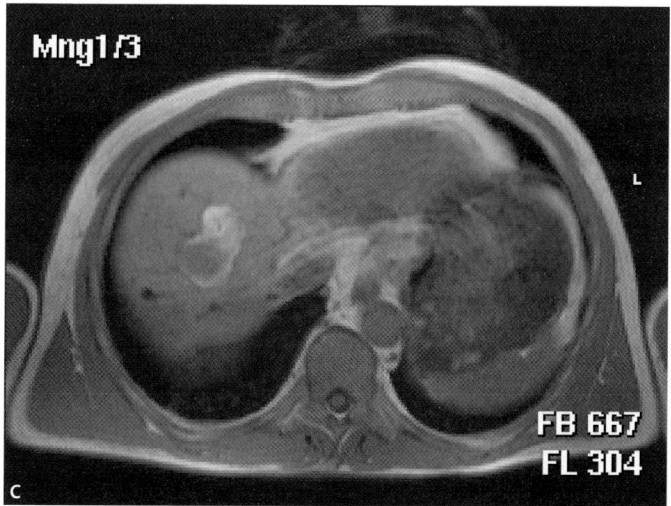

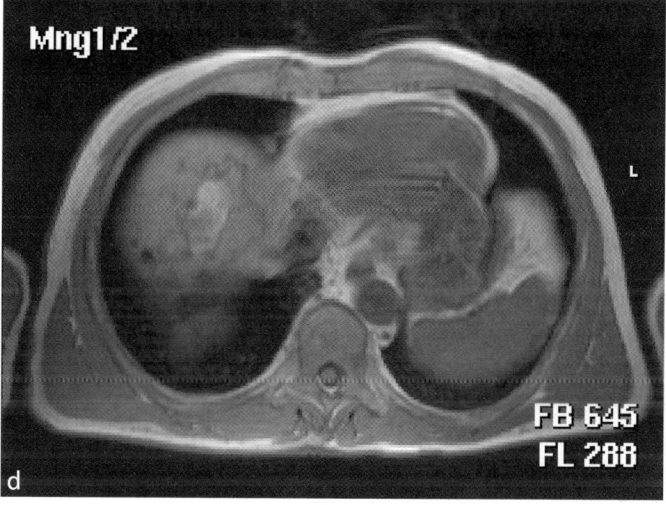

evidence of both intra- and extrahepatic spread. Initial results indicate that PET/CT imaging may prove to be more accurate when evaluating the ablative zone for residual tumor than image analysis based on morphologic data alone.

PET/CT may be expected to play a distinctive role in follow-up of patients undergoing RFA of liver lesions for the detection of residual unablated tumor. The advantages of fused PET/CT data sets over PET alone and CT alone are related to accurate localization of focally increased glucose metabolism in terms of therapeutic planning in an area of residual tumor, offering guidance of subsequent interventional procedures to these areas of viable tumor cells [31, 32].

6.4 Patient Outcome

The early clinical studies of RFA were performed in order to assess feasibility aiming at safety, tolerability, and local therapeutic effect of the treatment. During recent years, RFA has evolved significantly concerning technical developments and procedure-related improvements. Therefore, data collected in early studies may not be comparable with recent series. Beside a high number of published studies and recommendations for the standardization and reporting criteria in RFA studies, the analysis of clinical results of percutaneous radiofrequency ablation in liver metastases is still hampered by several problems [33]. Many reports presented data that involve different tumor entities, including primary and metastatic liver tumors with different tumor sizes. Treatment was performed with different types of RF generators and needle designs and additional therapies such as resection, regional or systemic chemotherapy, and other local ablative techniques have been used in combination to RFA. Finally, the studies have different endpoints and follow-up durations, as well as criteria for evaluating results.

6.4.1 Radiofrequency Ablation

In early clinical series, Solbiati et al. [34] and Lencioni et al. [35] performed RFA in patients with limited hepatic metastatic disease, who were excluded from surgery. In the first series, 29 patients with 44 hepatic metastases ranging from 1.3 to 5.1 cm in diameter were treated. Each tumor was treated in one or two sessions, and technical success, defined as the lack of residual unablated tumor at CT or MR imaging obtained 7–14 days after completion of treatment, was achieved in 40 of 44 lesions. However, follow-up imaging studies confirmed complete necrosis of the entire metastasis in only 66% of the cases, whereas local tumor progression was observed in the remaining 34%. Only one complication, self-limited hemorrhage, was seen. One-year survival was 94%. In the study by Lencioni et al. [35], 29 patients with 53 hepatic metastases ranging from 1.1 to 4.8 cm in diameter were enrolled. A total of 127 insertions were performed (mean, 2.4 insertions/lesion) during 84 treatment sessions (mean, 1.6 sessions/lesion) with no complications. Complete tumor response, defined as the presence of an unenhancing ablation zone larger than the treated tumor on posttreatment spiral CT, was seen in 41 (77%) of 53 lesions. After a mean follow-up period of 6.5 months (range, 3–9 months), local tumor progression was seen in 12% of cases. One-year survival was 93%. A systematic review on the outcomes of RFA for unresectable hepatic metastases in 2002 revealed a dearth of long-term follow-up data. Seidenfeld et al. [36] found only seven articles that provided data on disease-free or recurrence-free survival, rates of hepatic relapse, and median or percent survival at 1–5 years after treatment. Five studies reported 86%–94% survival at 1 year, but only one study reported survival at 2 years or longer [37]. In a recent study by Solbiati et al. [27], the results from 109 patients with 172 metastatic lesions who underwent RFA under ultrasound guidance were analyzed. The median follow-up was 3 years and local tumor control was achieved in 70% of the lesions. Local recurrence – including residual tumor foci – occurred in 30%, who were again treated by RFA so that the entire rate of local tumor control reached 78%. New metastases developed in 50.4% of the patients at a median time to recurrence of 12 months after RFA. The overall 2- and 3-year survival rates were 67% and 33%, respectively, and the median survival was 30 months. This compares favorably with data reported by Gillams et al. [10], with a median survival of 34 months and a 3-year survival of 36%. Survival of 36% at 3 years in inoperable patients is similar to patients undergoing resection for operable metastatic disease showing a 3-year survival of 42%–44% [38, 39]. In another larger series, 328 hepatic metastases in 76 patients were treated with RFA. At a mean follow-up of 15 months, local recurrence was noted in 9% [40]. Very recent data of the TRAIN study – Tumor Radiofrequency Ablation Italian Network by Lencioni et al. [1] – demonstrated long-term data on colorectal and breast cancer metastases to the liver treated by RFA. In colorectal metastases, 423 patients were evaluated presenting unifocal liver metastases (mean size, 2.7 cm). The overall survival after 1, 3, and 5 years was 86%, 47%, and 24%, respectively. Interestingly, they found a very good 5-year survival rate of 56% in a subgroup of patients having one tumor nodule equal or less than 2.5 cm in size. Patients with tumors bigger than 2.5 cm and multifocal tumors showed a significant decrease in the 5-year survival of 13% and 11%, respectively. Data of the 102 patients suffering from breast cancer metastases confirmed that in selected breast cancer patients where the metastases are unifocal with a mean diameter of 2.4 cm with no further extrahepatic spread, RFA plays an interesting role in the treatment strategy, with overall survival rates after 1, 3, and 5 years of 95%, 50%, and 30%, respectively [1] (Table 6.2).

6.4.2 Radiofrequency Ablation and Resection

Abdalla et al. [41] evaluated the role of RFA with respect to surgical resection. Survival of 418 patients with colorectal metastases isolated to the liver who were treated with hepatic resection (n = 190), RFA plus resection (n = 101), RFA

Table 6.2 Survival after RFA, selected references

Author	Patients	Tumor	Survival		
			1 year	3 years	5 years
Solbiati et al. 1997 [34]	29	CRC = 22	94%	–	–
Lencioni et al. 1998 [35]	29	CRC = 24	93%	–	–
Gillams et al. 2000 [50]	69	CRC	90%	34%	4 years: 22%
Solbiati et al. 2001 [27]	109	CRC	–	33%	–
Oshowo et al. 2003 [42]	25	CRC	–	52%	–
Abdalla et al. 2004 [41]	57	CRC	–	–	4a: 22%
Gillams et al. 2004 [9]	167	CRC	–	–	30%
Lencioni et al. 2004 [1]	423	CRC	86%	47%	24%
		CRC < 2.5 cm	–	–	56%
		CRC > 2.5 cm	–	–	13%
		CRC multifocal	–	–	11%
	102	Breast	95%	50%	30%

only (n = 57), or chemotherapy only (n = 70) was examined. Overall survival for patients treated with RFA plus resection or RFA only was greater than for those who received chemotherapy only (p = 0.0017). However, overall survival was highest after resection: 4-year survival rates after resection, RFA plus resection, and RFA only were 65%, 36%, and 22%, respectively (p< 0.0001). However, RFA only had been used only in patients where surgery was not possible and therefore could not be compared subsequently. In contrast, Oshowo et al. [42] showed no difference in survival outcome of patients with solitary colorectal liver metastases treated by surgery (n = 20) or by RFA (n = 25). In this study, the survival rate at 3 years was 55% for patients treated with surgery and 52% for RFA, suggesting that the survival after resection and RFA is equal. Elias et al. [43] demonstrated that RFA instead of repeated resections for the treatment of liver tumor recurrence after partial hepatectomy has the potential to increase the percentage of curative local treatments for liver recurrence after hepatectomy from 17% to 26% and to decrease the proportion of repeated hepatectomies from 100% to 39%. A completely different approach was done by Livraghi et al. [44]. They evaluated 88 patients with 134 colorectal liver metastases who were potential candidates for surgery concerning the potential role of performing RFA during the interval between diagnosis and resection as part of a "test-of-time" management approach. Among the 53 patients in whom complete tumor ablation was achieved after RF treatment, 98% were excluded from surgical resection: 44% because they remained free of disease and 56% because they developed additional metastases leading to unresectability. No patient in whom RF treatment did not achieve complete tumor ablation became unresectable due to the growth of the treated metastases.

6.4.3 Complications

A recent paper by Mulier et al. [45] reviewed the world literature until the end of 2001 concerning complications after radiofrequency ablation. A total of 3,670 patients were analyzed, including 2,898 patients having had a percutaneous approach for RFA. Mortality was found to be 0.5%, with sepsis, liver failure, and cardiac complications being the most important ones. De Baere et al. [46] reported a mortality rate of 1.4%, with portal vein thrombosis being responsible for the highest number of fatal outcomes. The entire complication rate of 10.6% is comparable to 7.2% presented by Mulier et al. [45]. In detail, Mulier et al. [45] reported intraperitoneal bleeding in 0.8%, subcapsular hematoma in 0.6%, biliary tract damage in 0.6%, pulmonary complications in 0.6%, pad skin burns in 0.6%, visceral damage in 0.5%, liver failure in 0.4%, hepatic vascular damage in 0.4%, and cardiac complications in 0.3%. A crucial fact with a high impact on potential treatment planning is reported by de Baere et al. [46], who showed that abscess occurred significantly more frequently in patients bearing a bilioenteric anastomosis, which was confirmed by the data of Livraghi et al. [11]. Seeding was shown to have a rate of 0.3% reported by Mulier et al. [45] in contrast to 12.5% from Llovet et al. [47], whereas de Baere et al. [46] also reported seeding to be rare, with 0.5%. The reason for this significant difference was most likely due to the technique used, with no track ablation. In a very recent multicenter study including 1,314 patients with 2542 HCC nodules by Livraghi et al. [48], neoplastic seeding was identified in 12 patients (0.9%); the rate was comparable at the three centres (0.9%, 0.7%, and 1.4%). Only previous biopsy was significantly associated with tumour seeding (p = 0.004). Although the authors included only HCC, it seems that the seeding rate reported by Llovet et al. [47] was definitely not representative concerning implantation metastases. Jaskolka et al. [49] found three statistically significant risk factors for needle tract seeding in 200 patients treated 298 times with RFA for different hepatic tumors: treatment of a subcapsular lesion (OR = 11.57, p = .007), multiple treatment sessions (OR = 2.0, p = .037), and multiple electrode placements (OR = 1.4, p = .006). Minor complications according to the SIR guidelines are usually not listed in the published data, so that the true (whenever clinically not relevant) complication rate may be even higher. Some late complications, such as bile duct strictures and electrode track seeding, may have been missed because of the short follow-up time in many studies.

6.5 Conclusions

Percutaneous RFA is an emerging minimally invasive procedure in patients suffering from non-resectable liver tumors, with survival rates for inoperable patients reaching the rates of patients undergoing resection. The effective and reproducible tumor destruction comes along with an acceptable mortality and morbidity. Although usually unfavorable patients in a highly palliative situation are treated with RFA, local tumor control by RFA is often equal to or even better than systemic chemotherapy. Combination of RFA with other treatments is an area of ongoing active research. It is highly desirable to implement local ablative therapies such as RFA in the treatment algorithm for nonresectable liver metastases, not only as third- but second-line treatment, probably in combination with systemic chemotherapy. RFA should always be embedded in a multidisciplinary treatment strategy tailored to the individual patient and to the features of the disease (customized therapy). Patient selection is very crucial for successful treatment with RFA. It should be based upon location, tumor size, proximity of large vessels, bleeding risk, respiratory motion, probe pathway, and of course the physician's experience. The technique is operator-dependent with a steep learning curve. Until the role of RFA within a multimodal treatment strategy for liver metastases has been completely defined, RFA should be restricted to centers with highly experienced interventionists incorporated into an interdisciplinary oncological team.

Because follow-up imaging is crucial in determining therapy success, imaging of ablation should also be performed by physicians experienced with RFA. To further assess the role of RFA in oncological patients, multicenter trials, more long-term follow-up data, further refinements in technique and procedure-related features, and studies of combined treatments including all therapies available for metastatic disease in the liver – all underway – must be evaluated with respect to the therapeutic reference standard to date.

References

1. Lencioni R, Crocetti L, Cioni D, Della Pina C, Bartolozzi C (2004) Percutaneous radiofrequency ablation of hepatic colorectal metastases: technique, indications, results, and new promises. Invest Radiol 39:689–697
2. Landis SH, Murray T, Bolden S, Wingo PA (1999) Cancer statistics, 1999. CA Cancer J Clin 49:8–31
3. Choti MA, Bulkley GB (1999) Management of hepatic metastases. Liver Transplant Surg 5:65–80
4. Scheele J, Altendorf-Hofmann A, Grube T, Hohenberger W, Stangl R, Schmidt K (2001) Resection of colorectal liver metastases. What prognostic factors determine patient selection? Chirurg 72:547–560
5. Redaelli CA, Dufour JF, Wagner M, Schilling M, Hüsler J, Krähenbühl L, Büchler MW, Reichen J (2002) Preoperative galactose elimination capacity predicts complications and survival after hepatic resection. Ann Surg 235:77–85
6. Ott R, Wein A, Hohenberger W (2001) Liver metastases – primary or multimodal therapy? Chirurg 71:887–897
7. Topham C, Adam R (2002) Oncosurgery: a new reality in metastatic colorectal carcinoma. Semin Oncol 29 [Suppl 15]:3–10
8. Hurwitz H, Fehrenbacher L, Novotny W, Cartwright T, Hainsworth J, Heim W, Berlin J, Baron A, Griffing S, Holmgren E, Ferrara N, Fyfe G, Rogers B, Ross R, Kabbinavar F (2004) Bevacizumab plus irinotecan, fluorouracil, and leucovorin for metastatic colorectal cancer. N Engl J Med 350:2335–2342
9. Gillams AR, Lees WR (2004) Radio-frequency ablation of colorectal liver metastases in 167 patients. Eur Radiol 14:2261–2267
10. Gillams A (2001) Thermal ablation of liver metastases. Abdominal Imaging 26:361–368
11. Livraghi T, Solbiati L, Meloni MF, Gazelle GS, Halpern EF, Goldberg SN (2003) Treatment of focal liver tumors with percutaneous radio-frequency ablation: complications encountered in a multicenter study. Radiology 226:441–451

12. Kainuma O, Asano T, Aoyama H, Takayama W, Nakagohri T, Kenmochi T, Hasegawa M, Tokoro Y, Sasagawa S, Ochiai T (1999) Combined therapy with radiofrequency thermal ablation and intra-arterial infusion chemotherapy for hepatic metastases from colorectal cancer. Hepatogastroenterology 46:1071–1077
13. Solbiati L, Ierace T, Goldberg SN, Sironi S, Livraghi T, Fiocca R, Servadio G, Rizzatto G, Mueller PR, Del Maschio A, Gazelle GS (1997) Percutaneous US-guided radio-frequency tissue ablation of liver metastases: treatment and follow-up in 16 patients. Radiology 202:195–203
14. McGahan JP, Dodd GD III (2001) Radiofrequency ablation of the liver: current status. Am J Roentgenol 176:3–16
15. Chen MH, Yang W, Yan K, Zou MW, Solbiati L, Liu JB, Dai Y (2004) Large liver tumors: protocol for radiofrequency ablation and its clinical application in 110 patients – mathematic model, overlapping mode, and electrode placement process. Radiology 232:260–271
16. Dodd GD 3rd, Frank MS, Aribandi M, Chopra S, Chintapalli KN (2001) Radiofrequency thermal ablation: computer analysis of the size of the thermal injury created by overlapping ablations. AJR Am J Roentgenol 177:777–782
17. Gillams AR (2005) The use of radiofrequency in cancer. Br J Cancer 92:1825–1829
18. Atwell TD, Charboneau JW, Que FG, Rubin J, Lewis BD, Nagorney DM, Callstrom MR, Farrell MA, Pitot HC, Hobday TJ (2005) Treatment of neuroendocrine cancer metastatic to the liver: the role of ablative techniques. Cardiovasc Intervent Radiol 228:409–421
19. Dromain C, de Baere T, Elias D, Kuoch V, Ducreux M, Boige V, Petrow P, Roche A, Sigal R (2002) Hepatic tumors treated with percutaneous radio-frequency ablation: CT and MR imaging follow-up. Radiology 223:255–262
20. Lim HK, Choi D, Lee WJ, Kim SH, Lee SJ, Jang HJ, Lee JH, Lim JH, Choo IW (2001) Hepatocellular carcinoma treated with percutaneous radiofrequency ablation: evaluation with follow-up multiphase helical CT. Radiology 221:447–454
21. Limanond P, Zimmerman P, Raman SS, Kadell BM, Lu DS (2003) Interpretation of CT and MRI after radiofrequency ablation of hepatic malignancies. Am J Roentgenol 181:1635–1640
22. Goldberg SN, Gazelle GS, Compton CC, Mueller PR, Tanabe KK (2000) Treatment of intrahepatic malignancy with radiofrequency ablation: radiologic–pathologic correlation. Cancer 88:2452–2463
23. Dupuy DE, Goldberg SN (2001) Image-guided radiofrequency tumor ablation: challenges and opportunities – Part II. J Vasc Interv Radiol 12:1135–1148
24. Choi H, Loyer EM, DuBrow RA, Kaur H, David CL, Huang S, Curley S, Charnsangavej C (2001) Radio-frequency ablation of liver tumors: assessment of therapeutic response and complications. RadioGraphics 21:S41–S54
25. Goldberg SN, Gazelle GS, Compton CC, Mueller PR, Tanabe KK (2000) Treatment of intrahepatic malignancy with radiofrequency ablation: radiologic–pathologic correlation. Cancer 88:2452–2463
26. Sironi S, Livraghi T, Meloni F, DeCobelli F, Ferero CG, Del Maschio A (1999) Small hepatocellular carcinoma treated with percutaneous RF ablation: MR imaging follow-up. Am J Roentgenol 173:1225–1229
27. Solbiati L, Ierace T, Tonolini M, Osti V, Cova L (2001) Radiofrequency thermal ablation of hepatic metastases. Eur J Ultrasound 13:149–158
28. Lim HK, Han JK (2002) Hepatocellular carcinoma: evaluation of therapeutic response to interventional procedures. Abdom Imaging 27:168–179
29. Tacke J (2003) Percutaneous radiofrequency ablation – clinical indications and results. Fortschr Roentgenstr 175:156–168
30. Pereira PL, Clasen S, Boss A, Schmidt D, Gouttefangeas C, Burkart C, Wiskirchen J, Tepe G, Claussen CD (2004) Radiofrequency ablation of liver metastases. Radiologe 44:347–357
31. Veit P, Antoch G, Stergar H, Bockisch A, Forsting M, Kuehl H (2005) Detection of residual tumor after radiofrequency ablation of liver metastasis with dual-modality PET/CT: initial results. Eur Radiol 16:80–87
32. Barker DW, Zagoria RJ, Morton KA, Kavanagh PV, Shen P (2005) Evaluation of liver metastases after radiofrequency ablation: utility of 18F-FDG PET and PET/CT. Am J Roentgenol 184:1096–1102

33. Goldberg SN, Grassi CJ, Cardella JF, Charboneau JW, Dodd III GD, Dupuy DE, Gervais D, Gillams AR, Kane RA, Lee FT Jr, Livraghi T, McGahan J, Phillips DA, Rhim H, Silverman SG, For the Society of Interventional Radiology Technology Assessment Committee and the International Working Group on Image-Guided Tumor Ablation (2005) Image-guided tumor ablation: standardization of terminology and reporting criteria. Radiology 235:728–739
34. Solbiati L, Goldberg SN, Ierace T, Livraghi T, Meloni F, Dellanoce M, Sironi S, Gazelle GS (1997) Hepatic metastases: percutaneous radio-frequency ablation with cooled-tip electrodes. Radiology 205:367–373
35. Lencioni R, Goletti O, Armillotta N, Paolicchi A, Moretti M, Cioni D, Donati F, Cicorelli A, Ricci S, Carrai M, Conte PF, Cavina E, Bartolozzi C (1998) Radio-frequency thermal ablation of liver metastases with a cooled-tip electrode needle: results of a pilot clinical trial. Eur Radiol 8:1205–1211
36. Seidenfeld J, Korn A, Aronson N (2002) Radiofrequency ablation of unresectable liver metastases. J Am Coll Surg 195:378–386
37. Solbiati L, Ierace T, Goldberg SN, Sironi S, Livraghi T, Fiocca R, Servadio G, Rizzatto G, Mueller PR, Del Maschio A, Gazelle GS (1997) Percutaneous US-guided radio-frequency tissue ablation of liver metastases: treatment and follow-up in 16 patients. Radiology 202:195–203
38. Jaeck D, Bachellier PGM, Boudjema K, Vaillant JC, Balladur P, Nordlinger B (1997) Long-term survival following resection of colorectal hepatic metastases. Association Française de Chirurgie. Br J Surg 84:977–980
39. Jenkins LT, Millikan KW, Bines SD, Staren ED, Doolas A (1997) Hepatic resection for metastatic colorectal cancer. Am Surg 63:605–610
40. Bowles BJ, Machi J, Limm WM, Severino R, Oishi AJ, Furumoto NL, Wong LL, Oishi RH (2001) Safety and efficacy of radiofrequency thermal ablation in advanced liver tumors. Arch Surg 136:864–869
41. Abdalla EK, Vauthey JN, Ellis LM, Ellis V, Pollock R, Broglio KR, Hess K, Curley SA (2004) Recurrence and outcomes following hepatic resection, radiofrequency ablation, and combined resection/ablation for colorectal liver metastases. Ann Surg 239:818–825; discussion 825–827
42. Oshowo A, Gillams A, Harrison E, Lees WR, Taylor I (2003) Comparison of resection and radiofrequency ablation for treatment of solitary colorectal liver metastases. Br J Surg 90:1240–1243
43. Elias D, De Baere T, Smayra T, Ouellet JF, Roche A, Lasser P (2002) Percutaneous radiofrequency thermoablation as an alternative to surgery for treatment of liver tumour recurrence after hepatectomy. Br J Surg 89:752–756
44. Livraghi T, Solbiati L, Meloni F, Ierace T, Goldberg SN, Gazelle GS (2003) Percutaneous radiofrequency ablation of liver metastases in potential candidates for resection: the "test-of-time approach". Cancer 97:3027–3035
45. Mulier S, Mulier P, Ni Y, Miao Y, Dupas B, Marchal G, De Wever I, Michel L (2002) Complications of radiofrequency coagulation of liver tumours. Br J Surg 89:1206–1222
46. De Baere T, Risse O, Kuoch V, Dromain C, Sengel C, Smayra T, El Din MG, Letoublon C, Elias D (2003) Adverse events during radiofrequency treatment of 582 hepatic tumors. AJR 181:695–700
47. Llovet JM, Vilana R, Bru C, Bianchi L, Salmeron JM, Boix L, Ganau S, Sala M, Pages M, Ayuso C, Sole M, Rodes J, Bruix J; Barcelona Clinic Liver Cancer (BCLC) Group (2001) Increased risk of tumor seeding after percutaneous radiofrequency ablation for single hepatocellular carcinoma. Hepatology 33:1124–1129
48. Livraghi T, Lazzaroni S, Meloni F, Solbiati L (2005) Risk of tumour seeding after percutaneous radiofrequency ablation for hepatocellular carcinoma. Br J Surg 92:856–858
49. Jaskolka JD, Asch MR, Kachura JR, Ho CS, Ossip M, Wong F, Sherman M, Grant DR, Greig PD, Gallinger S (2005) Needle tract seeding after radiofrequency ablation of hepatic tumors. J Vasc Interv Radiol 16:485–491
50. Gillams AR, Lees WR (2000) Survival after percutaneous, image-guided, thermal ablation of hepatic metastases from colorectal cancer. Dis Colon Rectum 43:656–661

7 Percutaneous Ablation of Hepatocellular Carcinoma

Riccardo Lencioni, Clodilde Della Pina, Laura Crocetti, Dania Cioni

7.1 Introduction

Hepatocellular carcinoma (HCC) is the fifth most common cancer, and its incidence is increasing worldwide because of the dissemination of hepatitis B and C virus infection. Patients with cirrhosis are at the highest risk of developing HCC and should undergo surveillance programs to detect the tumor at an early, asymptomatic stage (Bruix et al. 2001). Patients with early-stage HCC – as defined by the Barcelona-Clinic Liver Cancer staging classification (Bruix and Llovet 2002) – should be first considered for surgical treatment options, which may achieve 60%–70% 5-year survival in well-selected patients (Llovet et al. 2003). Hepatic resection is best indicated for patients with a single tumor and well-preserved liver function, who have neither abnormal bilirubin nor clinically relevant portal hypertension. However, less than 5% of cirrhotic patients with HCC fit these criteria (Llovet et al. 1999). Liver transplantation benefits patients who have decompensated cirrhosis and one tumor smaller than 5 cm or up to three nodules smaller than 3 cm each, but donor shortage greatly limits its applicability. This difficulty may be in part overcome by living donation, which, however, requires a highly skilled surgical team (Belghiti and Kianmanesch 2003; Schwartz 2004).

Advances in surgical techniques during the past two decades have led to effective treatment for selected patients with hepatic metastases. Surgical resection of colorectal cancer metastatic to the liver results in a 5-year survival rate of 40%, and liver metastases from other primary tumors, such as neuroendocrine carcinoma and genitourinary tumors, are also treated effectively with liver resection (Bentrem et al. 2005; Weitz et al. 2005). However, only 10%–25% of patients with metastases isolated to the liver are eligible for resection, because of extent and location of the disease or concurrent medical conditions (Lencioni et al. 2004b). Unfortunately, treatment of nonoperable or nonresectable patients with systemic or intra-arterial chemotherapy is not entirely satisfactory in terms of survival outcomes (Jonker et al. 2000).

Image-guided techniques for local tumor treatment have emerged as a viable therapeutic option for patients with limited hepatic malignant disease who are not surgical candidates. Over the past two decades, several methods for chemical ablation or thermal tumor destruction through localized heating or freezing have been developed and clinically tested (Table 7.1). While chemical and hyperthermic ablation techniques

Table 7.1 Percutaneous methods for ablation of hepatic neoplasms

Chemical ablation
Ethanol injection
Acetic acid injection
Thermal ablation
Radiofrequency ablation
Microwave ablation
Laser ablation
Cryoablation

have been widely performed via a percutaneous approach, most of the experience with cryotherapy has involved an open or laparoscopic approach. The present chapter focuses on the percutaneous use of chemical and hyperthermic ablation in the treatment of HCC and hepatic metastases.

7.2 Eligibility Criteria

A careful clinical, laboratory, and imaging assessment must be performed in each individual patient by a multidisciplinary team to evaluate eligibility for percutaneous ablation. Laboratory tests should include measurement of serum tumor markers, such as alpha-fetoprotein for HCC and carcinoembryonic antigen for colorectal metastases, as well as a full evaluation of the patient's coagulation status. A prothrombin time ratio (normal time/patient's time) greater than 50% and a platelet count higher than 50 000 platelets/µl are required to keep the risk of bleeding at an acceptably low level. The tumor staging protocol must be tailored to the type of malignancy. In patients with HCC, it should include abdominal ultrasound (US) and spiral computed tomography (CT) or dynamic magnetic resonance imaging (MRI), although in selected cases chest CT and bone scintigraphy may be needed to exclude extrahepatic tumor spread. Whole-body CT and positron emission tomography (PET) may be required to properly stage patients with hepatic metastases.

Percutaneous treatment is accepted as the best therapeutic choice for nonsurgical patients with early-stage HCC (Bruix et al. 2001; Lencioni et al. 2004a). Patients are required to have either a single tumor smaller than 5 cm or as many as three nodules smaller than 3 cm each, no evidence of vascular invasion or extrahepatic spread, performance status test of 0, and liver cirrhosis in Child-Pugh class A or B. In the setting of metastatic disease, percutaneous ablation is generally indicated for nonsurgical patients with colorectal cancer oligometastases isolated to the liver (Lencioni et al. 2004b; Gillams and Lees 2005). Selected patients with limited hepatic and pulmonary colorectal metastatic disease, however, may qualify for percutaneous treatment (Lencioni et al. 2004c; Berber et al. 2005). In patients with hepatic metastases from other primary cancers, promising initial results have been reported in the treatment of breast and endocrine tumors (Liang et al. 2003; Abe et al. 2005). The number of lesions should not be considered an absolute contraindication to percutaneous ablation if successful treatment of all metastatic deposits can be accomplished. Nevertheless, most centers preferentially treat patients with four or fewer lesions. Tumor size is of utmost importance to predict the outcome of percutaneous ablation. Imaging studies underestimate the size of metastatic deposits. Therefore, the target tumor should not exceed 3–4 cm in its longest axis to ensure complete ablation with most of the currently available devices.

Pretreatment imaging must carefully define the location of each lesion with respect to surrounding structures. Lesions located along the surface of the liver can be considered for percutaneous ablation, although their treatment requires adequate expertise and may be associated with a higher risk of complications. Thermal ablation of superficial lesions that are adjacent to any part of the gastrointestinal tract must be avoided because of the risk of thermal injury of the gastric or bowel wall (Rhim et al. 2004). The colon appears to be at greater risk than the stomach or small bowel for thermally mediated perforation. Gastric complications are rare, likely owing to the relatively greater wall thickness of the stomach or the rarity of surgical adhesions along the gastrohepatic ligament. The mobility of the small bowel may also provide the bowel with greater protection compared with the relatively fixed colon. A laparoscopy approach or the use of special techniques, such as intraperitoneal injection of dextrose to displace the bowel, can be considered in such instances. Treatment of lesions adjacent to the gallbladder or to the hepatic hilum is at risk of thermal injury of the biliary tract. In experienced hands, thermal ablation of tumors located in the vicinity of the gallbladder was shown to be feasible, although associated in most cases with self-limited iatrogenic cholecystitis (Chopra et al. 2003). In contrast, thermal ablation of lesions adjacent to hepatic vessels is possible, since flowing blood usually protects the vascular wall from thermal injury: in these cases, however, the risk of incomplete treatment of the neoplastic tissue close to the vessel may increase because of the heat loss by convection. The potential risk of thermal damage to critical structures should be weighted against benefits on a case-by-case basis.

7.3 Chemical Ablation

The seminal technique used for local ablation of hepatic tumors is percutaneous ethanol injection (PEI). Ethanol induces coagulation necrosis of the lesion as a result of cellular dehydration, protein denaturation, and chemical occlusion of small tumor vessels. PEI is a well-established technique for the treatment of nodular-type HCC. HCC nodules have a soft consistency and are surrounded by a firm cirrhotic liver. Consequently, injected ethanol diffuses within them easily and selectively, leading to complete necrosis of about 70% of small lesions (Shiina et al. 1991). An alternate method for chemical ablation is acetic acid injection. Although acetic acid injection has been reported to increase the success rate of PEI, this technique has been used by very few investigators worldwide. PEI – as well as other methods of chemical ablation – is not effective in the treatment of metastatic lesions. As opposed to HCC, ethanol diffusion within hepatic metastases is uneven, resulting in largely incomplete ablation with necrotic areas and viable tissue irregularly mixed (Livraghi et al. 1991).

7.3.1 Ethanol Injection

PEI is best administered by using US guidance because US allows for continuous real-time monitoring of the injection. This is crucial to realize the pattern of tumor perfusion and to avoid excessive ethanol leakage outside the lesion. Fine noncutting needles, with either a single end hole or multiple side holes, are commonly used for PEI. PEI is usually performed under local anesthesia and does not require patient hospitalization. The treatment schedule includes four to six sessions performed once or twice weekly. The number of treatment sessions, as well as the amount of injected ethanol per session, may vary greatly according to the size of the lesion, the pattern of tumor perfusion, and the compliance of the patient.

Although there have not been any prospective randomized trials comparing PEI and best supportive care or PEI and surgical resection, several retrospective studies have provided indirect evidence that PEI improves the natural history of HCC: the long-term outcomes of patients with small tumors who were treated with PEI were similar to those reported in surgical series, with 5-year survival rates ranging from 41% to 53% in Child A patients (Table 7.2). Of importance, two cohort studies and one retrospective case–control study comparing surgical resection and PEI failed to identify any difference in survival, even though patients in PEI groups had poorer liver function (Table 7.3). These data show that PEI is a useful treatment for patients with early-stage HCC and suggest that surgical resection may achieve better results only after strict candidate selection.

Although PEI is a low-risk procedure, severe complications have been reported. In a multicenter survey including 1,066 patients, one death (0.1%) and 34 complications (3.2%) – including seven cases of tumor seeding (0.7%) – were reported (Di Stasi et al. 1997). The major limitation of PEI is the high local recurrence rate, which may reach 33% in lesions smaller than 3 cm and 43% in lesions exceeding 3 cm (Khan et al. 2000; Koda et al. 2000). The injected ethanol does not always accomplish complete tumor necrosis because of its inhomogeneous distribution within the lesion – especially in presence of intratumoral septa – and the limited effect on extracapsular cancerous spread. Moreover, PEI is unable to create a safety margin of ablation in the liver parenchyma surrounding the nodule, and therefore may not destroy tiny satellite lesions which, even in small tumors, may be located in close proximity of the main nodule.

Injection of large volumes of ethanol in a single session performed under general anesthesia has been reported to enable successful PEI treatment of large or infiltrating HCC (Livraghi et al. 1998). However, results of single-session PEI are based on uncontrolled investigations and when critically compared with data on the natural

Table 7.2 Studies reporting long-term survival outcomes of patients with early-stage hepatocellular carcinoma who underwent percutaneous ethanol injection

Author and year	No. of patients	Survival rates (%)		
		1-year	3-year	5-year
Shiina et al. 1993	98	85	62	52
Lencioni et al. 1995	105	96	68	32
Livraghi et al. 1995				
Child A, single HCC <5 cm	293	98	79	47
Child B, single HCC <5 cm	149	93	63	29
Ryu et al. 1997				
Stage I, 1–3 HCC <3 cm[a]	110	98	84	54
Stage II, 1–3 HCC <3 cm[a]	140	91	65	45
Lencioni et al. 1997				
Child A, 1 HCC <5 cm or 3 <3 cm	127	98	79	53
Child B, 1 HCC <5 cm or 3 <3 cm	57	88	50	28
Pompili et al. 2001				
Child A, 1–2 HCC <5 cm	111	94	62	41
Teratani et al. 2002				
Age <70 years	516	90	65	40
Age >70 years	137	83	52	27

HCC, hepatocellular carcinoma
[a] Clinical stage according to the Liver Cancer Study Group of Japan

history and prognosis of untreated nonsurgical HCC, the benefits of the procedure are not evident.

7.3.2 Acetic Acid Injection

Acetic acid injection has been proposed as a viable alternative to PEI for the treatment of HCC. Two studies compared acetic acid injection and PEI. In the first paper, 60 patients with small HCC lesions were entered into a randomized trial. The 1- and 2-year survival rates were 100% and 92%, respectively, in the acetic acid injection group; and 83% and 63%, respectively, in the PEI group. A multivariate analysis of prognostic factors showed that treatment was an independent predictor of survival (Ohnishi et al. 1998). In contrast, in a prospective comparative study including 63 patients treated by acetic acid injection and 62 patients treated by PEI, no significant survival differences were observed between the two treatment groups (Huo et al. 2003). In summary, this alternate option for chemical ablation had limited diffusion and was not tested in large series of patients. The reported survival outcomes are not better than those obtained by several authors with PEI.

7.4 Thermal Ablation

Application of localized heating or freezing enables in situ destruction of malignant liver tumors preserving normal liver parenchyma. The thermal ablative therapies involved in clinical practice can be classified as either hepatic hyperthermic treatments – including radiofrequency (RF) ablation, microwave ablation, and laser ablation – or hepatic cryotherapy. Hepatic

Table 7.3 Studies comparing surgical resection and percutaneous ethanol injection in the treatment of early-stage hepatocellular carcinoma

Author and year	No. of patients	Survival rates (%)			P
		1-year	3-year	5-year	
Castells et al. 1993[a]					NS
Surgical resection	33	81	44	NA	
PEI	30	83	55	NA	
Yamamoto et al. 2001[a]					NS
Surgical resection	58	97	84	61	
PEI	39	100	82	59	
Daniele et al. 2003[b]					NS
Surgical resection	17	82	63	NA	
PEI	65	91	65	NA	

PEI, percutaneous ethanol injection; NA, not available; NS, not significant
[a] Cohort study
[b] Retrospective case-control study

hyperthermic treatments are mostly performed via a percutaneous approach, while an open or laparoscopic approach has been widely adopted for hepatic cryotherapy. This chapter focuses on percutaneous hyperthermic ablation in the treatment of HCC and hepatic metastases.

The thermal damage caused by heating is dependent on both the tissue temperature achieved and the duration of heating. Heating of tissue at 50°–55 °C for 4–6 min produces irreversible cellular damage. At temperatures between 60 °C and 100 °C, nearly immediate coagulation of tissue is induced, with irreversible damage to mitochondrial and cytosolic enzymes of the cells. At more than 100°–110 °C, tissue vaporizes and carbonizes (Goldberg et al. 2000). For adequate destruction of tumor tissue, the entire target volume must be subjected to cytotoxic temperatures. Different physical mechanisms are involved in the hepatic hyperthermic treatments in order to generate a lethal temperature. RF ablation is based on the interaction of an alternating electric current with living tissue. At a high-frequency setting (460–480 kHz), the current will cause agitation of ions in the adjacent tissue, which generate frictional heat that extends into the tissue by conduction. Microwave ablation relies on high-frequency electromagnetic radiation that is generated to heat the intracellular water molecules of the surrounding tissue. The resulting heat energy will lead to irreversible cellular damage. Laser ablation consists of a coherent, monochromatic and highly collimated beam of light. Focusing such light energy into the liver tumor results in heat production and coagulation.

An important factor that affects the success of thermal ablation is the ability to ablate all viable tumor tissue and an adequate tumor-free margin. To achieve rates of local tumor recurrence with thermal ablation that are comparable to those obtained with hepatic resection, a 360°, 1-cm-thick tumor-free margin should be produced around each tumor (Goldberg et al. 2000). This cuff is necessary to assure that all microscopic invasions around the periphery of a tumor have been eradicated. Thus, the target diameter of an ablation must be ideally 2 cm larger than the diameter of the tumor that undergoes treatment. For example, a 5-cm ablation device can be used to treat a 3-cm-diameter tumor. Otherwise, multiple overlapping ablations have to be performed (Dodd et al. 2001).

Thermal ablation is usually performed under conscious sedation or general anesthesia with standard cardiac, pressure, and oxygen monitoring. The lesion can be targeted with US, CT, or MR imaging. The guidance system is chosen largely on the basis of operator preference and local availability of dedicated equipment such as CT fluoroscopy or open MR systems. A percutaneously inserted metallic coil can be placed during the proper phase of contrast enhancement as a target to facilitate ablation of tumors poorly seen on CT or US (Adam et al. 2004). During the procedure, important aspects to be monitored include how well the tumor is being covered and whether any adjacent normal structures are being affected at the same time. While the transient hyperechoic zone that is seen at US within and surrounding a tumor during and immediately after RF ablation can be used as a rough guide to the extent of tumor destruction, MR is currently the only imaging modality with validated techniques for real-time temperature monitoring. To control an image-guided ablation procedure, the operator can utilize the image-based information obtained during monitoring or automated systems that terminate the ablation at a critical point in the procedure. At the end of the procedure, most systems allows the operator to ablate the needle track, which is aimed at preventing any tumor cell dissemination. Contrast-enhanced US performed after the end of the procedure may allow an initial evaluation of treatment effects. However, contrast-enhanced CT or MR imaging are recognized as the standard modalities to assess treatment outcome, although promising initial results have been reported by using PET. CT and MR images obtained after treatment show successful ablation as a nonenhancing area with or without a peripheral enhancing rim. The enhancing rim that may be observed along the periphery of the ablation zone appears as a relatively concentric, symmetric, and uniform process in an area with smooth inner margins. This is a transient finding that represents a benign physiologic response to thermal injury (initially, reactive hyperemia; subsequently, fibrosis and giant cell reaction). Benign periablational enhancement needs to be differentiated from irregular peripheral enhancement due to residual tumor that occurs at the treatment margin. In contrast to benign periablational enhancement, residual unablated tumor often grows in scattered, nodular, or eccentric patterns (Goldberg et al. 2003). Later follow-up imaging studies should be aimed at detecting the recurrence of the treated lesion (i.e., local tumor progression), the development of new hepatic lesions, or the emergence of extrahepatic disease.

7.4.1 Radiofrequency Ablation

The goal of RF ablation is to induce thermal injury to the tissue through electromagnetic energy deposition. The patient is part of a closed-loop circuit, which includes a RF generator, an electrode needle, and a large dispersive electrode (ground pads). An alternating electric field is created within the tissue of the patient. Because of the relatively high electrical resistance of tissue in comparison with the metal electrodes, there is marked agitation of the ions present in the target tissue that surrounds the electrode, since the tissue ions attempt to follow the changes in the direction of alternating electric current. The agitation results in frictional heat around the electrode. The discrepancy between the small surface area of the needle electrode and the large area of the ground pads causes the generated heat to be focused and concentrated around the needle electrode.

In the initial experience with RF treatment, a major limitation of the technique was the small volume of ablation created by conventional monopolar electrodes. These devices were capable of producing cylindrical ablation zones not greater than 1.6 cm in the short axis. Therefore, multiple electrode insertions were necessary to treat all but the smallest lesions. Subsequently, several strategies for increasing the ablation zone achieved with RF treatment have been used. Major progress was achieved with the introduction of modified electrodes, including internally cooled electrodes and multitined expandable electrodes (Goldberg et al. 2003). Internally cooled electrodes consist of dual-lumen electrodes with an exposed active tip of variable length. Internal cooling is obtained by continuous perfusion with chilled saline and is aimed at preventing overheating of tissues nearest the electrode to minimize carbonization and gas formation around the tip. Multitined expandable electrodes have an active surface that can be substantially increased by prongs deployed from the tip. In application, the tip of the needle is advanced to the target lesion and the curved electrodes are deployed into the tumor according to the desired volume of ablation.

Most early clinical research with RF ablation was conducted in the framework of feasibility studies, aimed at demonstrating the local effect and the safety of the procedure (Solbiati et al. 1997; Lencioni et al. 1998; Curley et al. 1999; Wood et al. 2000). More recently, the clinical efficacy of RF ablation has been evaluated in the treatment of HCC and colorectal hepatic metastases.

7.4.1.1 Treatment of Hepatocellular Carcinoma

RF ablation has been the most widely assessed alternative to PEI for local ablation of HCC. Histologic data from explanted liver specimens in patients who underwent RF ablation showed that tumor size and presence of large (3 mm or more) abutting vessels significantly affect the local treatment effect. Complete tumor necrosis was pathologically shown in 83% of tumors less than 3 cm and 88% of tumors in nonperivascular location (Lu et al. 2005). In two comparative studies, the rates of complete tumor response as shown by posttreatment CT were higher in patients who underwent RF ablation with respect to those submitted to PEI (Livraghi et al. 1999; Ikeda et al. 2001).

Two randomized studies compared RF ablation vs PEI for the treatment of early-stage HCC (Table 7.4). In the first trial, Child A or B patients with either a uninodular tumor less than 5 cm or as many as three tumors less than 3 cm each were randomly assigned to receive RF ablation or PEI (Lencioni et al. 2003). The overall survival rates at 1 and 2 years were 100% and 98%, respectively, in the RF group and 96% and 88%, respectively, in the PEI group. Despite the tendency favoring RF ablation, the observed difference did not reach statistical significance, likely because of the short follow-up period. However, 1- and 2-year recurrence-free survival rates were significantly higher in RF-treated patients than in PEI-treated patients, and RF treatment was confirmed as an independent prognostic factor for local recurrence-free survival by multivariate analysis (Lencioni et al. 2003). In the second study, patients with HCCs 4 cm or less were randomly assigned to three groups (conventional PEI group, higher-dose PEI group, and RF group) (Lin et al. 2004). The overall and the cancer-free survival rates were highest in the RF group, and multivariate analysis determined that tumor size, tumor differentiation, and the method of treatment (RF vs both methods of PEI) were significant factors in

Table 7.4 Randomized studies comparing radiofrequency ablation and percutaneous ethanol injection in the treatment of early-stage hepatocellular carcinoma

Author and year	No. of patients	Survival rates (%)			P
		1-year	2-year	3-year	
Lencioni et al. 2003					NS
Radiofrequency ablation	52	100	98	NA	
PEI	50	96	88	NA	
Lin et al. 2004					<0.05[a]
Radiofrequency ablation	50	90	82	74	
Conventional PEI	46	85	61	50	
Higher-dose PEI	50	88	63	55	

PEI, percutaneous ethanol injection; NA, not available; NS, not significant
[a] Radiofrequency ablation vs conventional PEI: P = 0.014, radiofrequency ablation vs higher-dose PEI: P = 0.02

relation to local tumor progression, overall survival, and cancer-free survival.

Two studies recently reported the long-term survival outcomes of RF ablation-treated patients (Table 7.5). In the first paper, 206 patients with early-stage HCC who were not candidates for resection or transplantation were enrolled in a prospective, intention-to-treat clinical trial (Lencioni et al. 2005a). RF ablation was considered as the first-line nonsurgical treatment and was actually performed in 187 (91%) of 206 patients. Nineteen (9%) of 206 patients had to be excluded from RF treatment because of the unfavorable location of the tumor. In patients who underwent RF ablation, survival depended on the severity of the underlying cirrhosis and the tumor multiplicity. Patients in Child class A had 3- and 5-year survival rates of 76% and 51%, respectively, while those in Child class B had 3- and 5-year survival rates of 46% and 31%, respectively. In the second study, 319 patients received RFA as primary treatment (naive patients) and 345 patients received RFA for recurrent tumor after previous treatment including resection, PEI, microwave ablation, and transarterial embolization (Tateishi et al. 2005). The cumulative survival rates at 3 and 5 years were 78% and 54%, respectively, for naive patients; and 62% and 38%, respectively, for nonnaive patients. Of interest, in a comparative study of RF ablation vs surgical resection in patients with a Child-Pugh score of 5 and a single HCC less than 4 cm in diameter, no differences in overall survival rates and cumulative recurrence-free survival rates were observed, despite a higher rate of local recurrence in the RF group (Hong et al. 2005).

Table 7.5 Studies reporting long-term survival outcomes of patients with early-stage hepatocellular carcinoma who underwent percutaneous radiofrequency ablation

Author and year	No. of patients	Survival rates (%)		
		1-year	3-year	5-year
Lencioni et al. 2005[a]				
Child A, 1 HCC < 5 cm or 3 < 3 cm	144	100	76	51
Child B, 1 HCC < 5 cm or 3 < 3 cm	43	89	46	31
Tateishi et al. 2005				
Naive patients[a]	319	95	78	54
Nonnaive patients[b]	345	92	62	38

HCC, hepatocellular carcinoma
[a] Patients who received radiofrequency ablation as primary treatment
[b] Patients who received radiofrequency ablation for recurrent tumor after previous treatment including resection, ethanol injection, microwave ablation, and transarterial embolization

Table 7.6 Studies reporting long-term survival outcomes of patients with colorectal hepatic metastases who underwent percutaneous radiofrequency ablation

Author and year	No. of patients	Survival rates (%)		
		1-year	3-year	5-year
Solbiati et al. 2001	117	93	46	NA
Lencioni et al., 2004a	423	86	47	24
Gillams et al. 2004	73	99	58	30

NA, not available

Despite the many published reports, some questions remain unanswered. Some authors have reported that RF ablation may be a safe and effective bridge to liver transplantation (Fontana et al. 2002; Wong et al. 2004). However, randomized studies would be needed to determine advantages and disadvantages of RF ablation with respect to transcatheter arterial chemoembolization for HCC patients awaiting transplantation. Recent studies have reported encouraging initial results in the treatment of large HCC lesions with a combination of RF ablation and balloon catheter occlusion of the tumor arterial supply or prior transcatheter arterial chemobolization (Yamasaki et al. 2002; Kitamoto et al. 2003; Lencioni et al. 2005b). However, further clinical trials are warranted to determine the survival impact of this approach.

7.4.1.2 Treatment of Hepatic Metastases

Many studies have investigated the use of RF ablation in the treatment of limited hepatic metastatic disease in patients who were excluded from surgery. Two early studies reported rates of complete response that did not exceed 60%–70% (Solbiati et al. 1997; Lencioni et al. 1998). Subsequently, owing to the advances in the RF technique, reported rates of successful local tumor control following RF treatment substantially increased. In two series, RF ablation allowed eradication of 91% of 100 metastases and 97% of 74 metastases (De Baere et al. 2000; Helmberger et al. 2001). Recently, data on long-term survival of nonsurgical patients with hepatic colorectal metastases who underwent RF ablation have been reported (Table 7.6). In particular, in two series including patients with five or fewer lesions, each 5 cm or less in diameter, the 5-year survival rate ranged from 24% to 30% at 5 years (Lencioni et al. 2004b; Gillams and Lees 2004). These figures are substantially higher than those obtained with any chemotherapy regimens and provide indirect evidence that RF ablation therapy improves survival in patients with limited hepatic metastatic disease.

Recent studies analyzed the role of RF ablation with respect to surgical resection. In one study, 418 patients with colorectal metastases isolated to the liver were treated with hepatic resection, RF ablation plus resection, RF ablation only, or chemotherapy only. Overall survival for patients treated with RF ablation plus resection or RF ablation only was greater than for those who received chemotherapy only. However, overall survival was highest after resection: 4-year survival rates after resection, RF ablation plus resection, and RF ablation only were 65%, 36%, and 22%, respectively (Abdalla et al. 2004). In another paper, the outcome of patients with solitary colorectal liver metastasis treated by surgery or by RF ablation did not differ: the survival rate at 3 years was 55% for patients treated with surgery and 52% for those who underwent RF ablation (Oshowo et al. 2003). Other authors used RF ablation instead of repeated resection for the treatment of liver tumor recurrence after partial hepatectomy (Elias et al. 2002). The potential role of performing RF ablation during the interval between diagnosis and resection as part of a "test-of-time" management approach was investigated (Livraghi et al. 2003a). Eighty-eight consecutive patients with colorectal liver metastases who were potential candidates for surgery were treated with RF ablation. Among the 53 patients in whom complete tumor ablation was achieved after RF treatment, 98% were spared surgical resection because they remained free of disease or because they developed additional metastases leading to unresectability. No patient in whom RF treatment did not achieve complete tumor ablation became unresectable due to the growth of the treated metastases.

7.4.1.3 Complications

Recently, three separate multicenter surveys have reported acceptable morbidity and mortality rates for a minimally invasive technique. The mortality rate ranged from 0.1% to 0.5%, the major complication rate ranged from 2.2% to 3.1%, and the minor complication rate ranged from 5% to 8.9% (Rhim et al. 2005). The most common causes of death were sepsis, hepatic failure, colon perforation, and portal vein thrombosis, while the most common complications were intraperitoneal bleeding, hepatic abscess, bile duct injury, hepatic decompensation, and grounding pad burns (Livraghi et al. 2003b; De Baere et al. 2003; Bleicher et al. 2003). Minor complications and side effects were usually transient and self-limiting. An uncommon late complication of RF ablation can be tumor seeding along the needle track. In patients with HCC, tumor seeding occurred in eight (0.5%) of 1610 cases in a multicenter survey (Livraghi et al. 2003b) and in one (0.5%) of 187 cases in a single-institution series (Lencioni et al. 2005a). Lesions with subcapsular location and an invasive tumoral pattern, as shown by a poor differentiation degree, seem to be at higher risk for such a complication (Llovet et al. 2001). While these data indicate that RF ablation is a relatively safe procedure, a careful assessment of the risks and benefits associated with the treatment must be made in each individual patient by a multidisciplinary team.

7.4.2 Microwave Ablation

"Microwave ablation" is the term used for all electromagnetic methods of inducing tumor destruction by using devices with frequencies greater than or equal to 900 kHz. The passage of microwaves into cells or other materials containing water results in the rotation of individual molecules. This rapid molecular rotation generates and uniformly distributes heat, which is instantaneous and continuous until the radiation is stopped. Microwave irradiation creates an ablation area around the needle in a column or round shape, depending on the type of needle used and the generating power (Lu et al. 2001).

Most clinical studies of microwave ablation investigated the usefulness of the technique in the treatment of HCC. The local effect of treatment was assessed in explanted livers by examining the histological changes of the tumor after microwave ablation. In one study, 89% of 18 small tumors were ablated completely (Yamashiki et al. 2003). Coagulative necrosis with faded nuclei and eosinophilic cytoplasm were the predominant findings in the ablated areas. There were also areas in which the tumors maintained their native morphological features as if the area were fixed, but their cellular activity was destroyed, as demonstrated by succinic dehydrogenase stain. One study compared microwave ablation and PEI in a retrospective evaluation of 90 patients with small HCC (Seki et al. 1999). The overall 5-year survival rates for patients with well-differentiated HCC treated with microwave ablation and PEI were not significantly different. However, among the patients with moderately or poorly differentiated HCC, overall survival with microwave ablation was significantly better than with PEI. In a large series including 234 patients, the 3- and 5-year survival rates were 73% and 57%, respectively (Dong et al. 2003). At a multivariate analysis, tumor size, number of nodules, and Child-Pugh classification had a significant effect on survival (Liang et al. 2005). Only one randomized trial compared the effectiveness of microwave ablation with that of RF ablation (Shibata et al. 2002). Seventy-two patients with 94 HCC nodules were randomly assigned to RF ablation and microwave ablation groups. Unfortunately, in this study the data were analyzed with respect to lesions and not to patients. Although no statistically significant differences were observed with respect to the efficacy of the two procedures, a tendency favoring RF ablation was recognized with respect to local recurrences and complications rates.

Limited data have been reported thus far concerning the use of microwave ablation in the treatment of hepatic metastases. In one study, 30 patients with multiple metastatic colorectal tumors in the liver who were potentially amenable to hepatic resection were randomly assigned to treatment with microwave coagulation (14 patients) or hepatectomy (16 patients). One- and 3-year survival rates and mean survival times were 71%, 14%, and 27 months, respectively, in the microwave group, whereas they were 69%, 23%, and 25 months, respectively, in the hepatectomy group (Shibata et al. 2000). The difference between these two groups was statistically not significant. Other authors have reported initial promising results in the treatment of hepatic metastases from other primary sites (Liang et al. 2003; Abe et al. 2005).

7.4.3 Laser Ablation

The term "laser ablation" should be used for ablation with light energy applied via fibers directly inserted into the tissue. A great variety of laser sources and wavelengths are available. In addition, different types of laser fibers, modified tips, and single or multiple laser applicators can be used. From a single, bare 400-μm laser fiber, a spherical volume of coagulative necrosis up to 2 cm in diameter can be produced. Use of higher power results in charring and vaporization around the fiber tip. Two methods have been developed for producing larger volumes of necrosis. The first consists of firing multiple bare fibers arrayed at 2-cm spacing throughout a target lesion, while the second uses cooled-tip diffuser fibers that can deposit up to 30 W over a large surface area, thus diminishing local overheating (Vogl et al. 1995).

To date, few data are available concerning the clinical efficacy of laser ablation. No randomized trials to compare laser ablation with any other treatment have been published thus far. In one study including 74 patients with early-stage HCC, overall survival rates were 68% at 3 years and 15% at 5 years, respectively (Pacella et al. 2001). Two single-institution series of patients with liver metastases from colorectal cancer who underwent laser ablation reported 5-year survival rates ranging from 4% to 37%, likely reflecting differences in equipment and inclusion criteria (Christophi et al. 2004; Vogl et al. 2004). Laser ablation appears to be relatively safe, with a major complication rate less than 2% (Vogl et al. 2002). The major drawback of current laser technology appears to be the small volume of ablation that can be created with a single-probe insertion. Insertion of multiple fibers is technically cumbersome and may not be feasible in lesions that are not conveniently located. New devices could overcome this limitation.

7.5 Conclusions

Several percutaneous techniques have been developed to treat nonsurgical patients with liver malignancies. These minimally invasive procedures can achieve effective and reproducible tumor destruction with acceptable morbidity. Percutaneous ablation is accepted as the best therapeutic choice for patients with early-stage HCC when resection or transplantation are precluded. PEI is the seminal technique for local ablation of HCC, and may achieve a 5-year survival rate of 50% in selected Child A patients. RF ablation constitutes the most assessed alternative technique. On the basis of the identified evidence, RF ablation seems to reach higher cumulative survival and recurrence-free survival rates compared with PEI. RF ablation has also become a viable treatment method for patients with limited hepatic metastatic disease from colorectal cancer who are not eligible for surgical resection. Further trials are needed to establish the clinical efficacy of the other percutaneous treatments. An appropriate use of percutaneous ablation techniques can only be done when the therapeutic strategy is decided by a multidisciplinary team and is tailored to the individual patient and to the features of the disease.

References

1. Abdalla EK, Vauthey JN, Ellis LM et al. (2004) Recurrence and outcomes following hepatic resection, radiofrequency ablation, and combined resection/ablation for colorectal liver metastases. Ann Surg 239:818–825
2. Abe H, Kurumi Y, Naka S et al. (2005) Open-configuration MR-guided microwave thermocoagulation therapy for metastatic liver tumors from breast cancer. Breast Cancer 12:26–31
3. Adam A, Hatzidakis A, Hamady M et al. (2004) Percutaneous coil placement prior to radiofrequency ablation of poorly visible hepatic tumors. Eur Radiol 14:1688–1691
4. Belghiti J, Kianmanesh R (2003) Surgical techniques used in adult living donor liver transplantation. Liver Transpl 9 [Suppl 2]:S29–S34
5. Bentrem DJ, Dematteo RP, Blumgart LH (2005) Surgical therapy for metastatic disease to the liver. Annu Rev Med 56:139–156
6. Berber E, Pelley R, Siperstein AE (2005) Predictors of survival after radiofrequency thermal ablation of colorectal cancer metastases to the liver: a prospective study. J Clin Oncol 23:1358–1364
7. Bleicher RJ, Allegra DP, Nora DT et al. (2003) Radiofrequency ablation in 447 complex unresectable liver tumors: lessons learned. Ann Surg Oncol 10:52–58
8. Bruix J, Llovet JM (2002) Prognostic prediction and treatment strategy in hepatocellular carcinoma. Hepatology 35:519–524

9. Bruix J, Sherman M, Llovet JM et al; EASL Panel of Experts on HCC (2001) Clinical management of hepatocellular carcinoma. Conclusions of the Barcelona-2000 EASL conference. European Association for the Study of the Liver. J Hepatol 35:421–430
10. Castells A, Bruix J, Bru C et al. (1993) Treatment of small hepatocellular carcinoma in cirrhotic patients: a cohort study comparing surgical resection and percutaneous ethanol injection. Hepatology 18:1121–1126
11. Chopra S, Dodd GD 3rd, Chanin MP, Chintapalli KN (2003) Radiofrequency ablation of hepatic tumors adjacent to the gallbladder: feasibility and safety. AJR Am J Roentgenol 180:697–701
12. Christophi C, Nikfarjam M, Malcontenti-Wilson C, Muralidharan V (2004) Long-term survival of patients with unresectable colorectal liver metastases treated by percutaneous interstitial laser thermotherapy. World J Surg 28:987–994
13. Curley SA, Izzo F, Delrio P et al. (1999) Radiofrequency ablation of unresectable primary and metastatic malignancies: results in 123 patients. Ann Surg 230:1–8
14. Daniele B, De Sio I, Izzo F et al; CLIP Investigators (2003) Hepatic resection and percutaneous ethanol injection as treatments of small hepatocellular carcinoma: a Cancer of the Liver Italian Program (CLIP 08) retrospective case–control study. J Clin Gastroenterol 36:63–67
15. De Baere T, Elias D, Dromain C et al. (2000) Radiofrequency ablation of 100 hepatic metastases with a mean follow-up of more than 1 year. AJR Am J Roentgenol 175:1619–1625
16. De Baere T, Risse O, Kuoch V et al. (2003) Adverse events during radiofrequency treatment of 582 hepatic tumors. AJR Am J Roentgenol 181:695–700
17. Di Stasi M, Buscarini L, Livraghi T et al. (1997) Percutaneous ethanol injection in the treatment of hepatocellular carcinoma. A multicenter survey of evaluation practices and complication rates. Scand J Gastroenterol 32:1168–1173
18. Dodd GD 3rd, Frank MS, Aribandi M et al. (2001) Radiofrequency thermal ablation: computer analysis of the size of the thermal injury created by overlapping ablations. AJR Am J Roentgenol 177:777–782
19. Dong B, Liang P, Yu X et al. (2003) Percutaneous sonographically guided microwave coagulation therapy for hepatocellular carcinoma: results in 234 patients. AJR Am J Roentgenol 180:1547–1555
20. Elias D, De Baere T, Smayra T et al. (2002) Percutaneous radiofrequency thermoablation as an alternative to surgery for treatment of liver tumour recurrence after hepatectomy. Br J Surg 89:752–756
21. Fontana RJ, Hamidullah H, Nghiem H et al. (2002) Percutaneous radiofrequency thermal ablation of hepatocellular carcinoma: a safe and effective bridge to liver transplantation. Liver Transpl 8:1165–1174
22. Gillams AR, Lees WR (2004) Radio-frequency ablation of colorectal liver metastases in 167 patients. Eur Radiol 14:2261–2267
23. Gillams AR, Lees WR (2005) Radiofrequency ablation of colorectal liver metastases. Abdom Imaging 30:419–426
24. Goldberg SN, Gazelle GS, Mueller PR (2000) Thermal ablation therapy for focal malignancies: a unified approach to underlying principles, techniques, and diagnostic imaging guidance. AJR Am J Roentgenol 174:323–331
25. Goldberg SN, Charboneau JW, Dodd GD 3rd et al. International Working Group on Image-Guided Tumor Ablation (2003) Image-guided tumor ablation: proposal for standardization of terms and reporting criteria. Radiology 228:335–345
26. Helmberger T, Holzknecht N, Schopf U et al. (2001) Radiofrequency ablation of liver metastases. Technique and initial results. Radiologe 41:69–76
27. Hong SN, Lee SY, Choi MS et al. (2005) Comparing the outcomes of radiofrequency ablation and surgery in patients with a single small hepatocellular carcinoma and well-preserved hepatic function. J Clin Gastroenterol 39:247–252
28. Huo TI, Huang YH, Wu JC et al. (2003) Comparison of percutaneous acetic acid injection and percutaneous ethanol injection for hepatocellular carcinoma in cirrhotic patients: a prospective study. Scand J Gastroenterol 38: 770–778
29. Ikeda M, Okada S, Ueno H et al. (2001) Radiofrequency ablation and percutaneous ethanol injection in patients with small hepatocellular carcinoma: a comparative study. Jpn J Clin Oncol 31:322–326

30. Jonker DJ, Maroun JA, Kocha W (2000) Survival benefit of chemotherapy in metastatic colorectal cancer: a meta-analysis of randomized controlled trials. Br J Cancer 82:1789–1794
31. Khan KN, Yatsuhashi H, Yamasaki K et al. (2000) Prospective analysis of risk factors for early intrahepatic recurrence of hepatocellular carcinoma following ethanol injection. J Hepatol 32:269–278
32. Kitamoto M, Imagawa M, Yamada H et al. (2003) Radiofrequency ablation in the treatment of small hepatocellular carcinomas: comparison of the radiofrequency effect with and without chemoembolization. AJR Am J Roentgenol 181:997–1003
33. Koda M, Murawaki Y, Mitsuda A et al. (2000) Predictive factors for intrahepatic recurrence after percutaneous ethanol injection therapy for small hepatocellular carcinoma. Cancer 88:529–537
34. Lencioni R, Bartolozzi C, Caramella D et al. (1995) Treatment of small hepatocellular carcinoma with percutaneous ethanol injection. Analysis of prognostic factors in 105 Western patients. Cancer 76:1737–1746
35. Lencioni R, Pinto F, Armillotta N et al. (1997) Long-term results of percutaneous ethanol injection therapy for hepatocellular carcinoma in cirrhosis: a European experience. Eur Radiol 7:514–519
36. Lencioni R, Goletti O, Armillotta N et al. (1998) Radio-frequency thermal ablation of liver metastases with a cooled-tip electrode needle: results of a pilot clinical trial. Eur Radiol 8:1205–1211
37. Lencioni R, Allgaier HP, Cioni D et al. (2003) Small hepatocellular carcinoma in cirrhosis: randomized comparison of radiofrequency thermal ablation versus percutaneous ethanol injection. Radiology 228:235–240
38. Lencioni R, Cioni D, Crocetti L, Bartolozzi C (2004a) Percutaneous ablation of hepatocellular carcinoma: state-of-the-art. Liver Transpl 10 [Suppl 1]:S91–S97
39. Lencioni R, Crocetti L, Cioni D et al. (2004b) Percutaneous radiofrequency ablation of hepatic colorectal metastases. Technique, indications, results, and new promises. Invest Radiol 39:689–697
40. Lencioni R, Crocetti L, Cioni R et al. (2004c) Radiofrequency ablation of lung malignancies: where do we stand? Cardiovasc Intervent Radiol 27:581–590
41. Lencioni R, Cioni D, Crocetti L et al (2005a) Early-stage hepatocellular carcinoma in cirrhosis: long-term results of percutaneous image-guided radiofrequency ablation. Radiology 234:961–967
42. Lencioni R, Della Pina C, Bartolozzi C (2005b) Percutaneous image-guided radiofrequency ablation in the therapeutic management of hepatocellular carcinoma. Abdom Imaging 30:401–408
43. Liang P, Dong B, Yu X et al. (2003) Prognostic factors for percutaneous microwave coagulation therapy of hepatic metastases. AJR Am J Roentgenol 181:1319–1325
44. Liang P, Dong B, Yu X et al. (2005) Prognostic factors for survival in patients with hepatocellular carcinoma after percutaneous microwave ablation. Radiology 235:299–307
45. Lin SM, Lin CJ, Lin CC et al. (2004) Radiofrequency ablation improves prognosis compared with ethanol injection for hepatocellular carcinoma ± 4 cm. Gastroenterology 127:1714–1723
46. Livraghi T, Vettori C, Lazzaroni S (1991) Liver metastases: results of percutaneous ethanol injection in 14 patients. Radiology 179:709–712
47. Livraghi T, Giorgio A, Marin G et al. (1995) Hepatocellular carcinoma and cirrhosis in 746 patients: long-term results of percutaneous ethanol injection. Radiology 197:101–108
48. Livraghi T, Benedini V, Lazzaroni S et al. (1998) Long-term results of single-session percutaneous ethanol injection in patients with large hepatocellular carcinoma. Cancer 83:48–57
49. Livraghi T, Goldberg SN, Lazzaroni S et al. (1999) Small hepatocellular carcinoma: treatment with radio-frequency ablation versus ethanol injection. Radiology 210:655–661
50. Livraghi T, Solbiati L, Meloni F et al. (2003a) Percutaneous radiofrequency ablation of liver metastases in potential candidates for resection: the "test-of-time approach". Cancer 97:3027–3035
51. Livraghi T, Solbiati L, Meloni MF et al. (2003b) Treatment of focal liver tumors with percutaneous radio-frequency ablation: complications encountered in a multicenter study. Radiology 226:441–451
52. Llovet JM, Fuster J, Bruix J (1999) Intention-to-treat analysis of surgical treatment for early hepatocellular carcinoma: resection versus transplantation. Hepatology 30:1434–1440

53. Llovet JM, Vilana R, Bru C et al. Barcelona Clinic Liver Cancer (BCLC) Group (2001) Increased risk of tumor seeding after percutaneous radiofrequency ablation for single hepatocellular carcinoma. Hepatology 33:1124–1129
54. Llovet JM, Burroughs A, Bruix J (2003) Hepatocellular carcinoma. Lancet 362:1907–1917
55. Lu DS, Yu NC, Raman SS et al. (2005) Radiofrequency ablation of hepatocellular carcinoma: treatment success as defined by histologic examination of the explanted liver. Radiology 234:954–960
56. Lu MD, Chen JW, Xie XY et al. (2001) Hepatocellular carcinoma: US-guided percutaneous microwave coagulation therapy. Radiology 221:167–172
57. Ohnishi K, Yoshioka H, Ito S, Fujiwara K (1998) Prospective randomized controlled trial comparing percutaneous acetic acid injection and percutaneous ethanol injection for small hepatocellular carcinoma. Hepatology 27:67–72
58. Oshowo A, Gillams A, Harrison E et al. (2003) Comparison of resection and radiofrequency ablation for treatment of solitary colorectal liver metastases. Br J Surg 90:1240–1243
59. Pacella CM, Bizzarri G, Magnolfi F et al. (2001) Laser thermal ablation in the treatment of small hepatocellular carcinoma: results in 74 patients. Radiology 221:712–720
60. Pompili M, Rapaccini GL, Covino M et al. (2001) Prognostic factors for survival in patients with compensated cirrhosis and small hepatocellular carcinoma after percutaneous ethanol injection therapy. Cancer 92:126–135
61. Rhim H (2005) Complications of radiofrequency ablation in hepatocellular carcinoma. Abdom Imaging 30:409–418
62. Rhim H, Dodd GD 3rd, Chintapalli KN et al. (2004) Radiofrequency thermal ablation of abdominal tumors: lessons learned from complications. Radiographics 24:41–52
63. Ryu M, Shimamura Y, Kinoshita T et al. (1997) Therapeutic results of resection, transcatheter arterial embolization and percutaneous transhepatic ethanol injection in 3225 patients with hepatocellular carcinoma: a retrospective multicenter study. Jpn J Clin Oncol 27:251–257
64. Schwartz M (2004) Liver transplantation for hepatocellular carcinoma. Gastroenterology 127 [Suppl 1]: S268–S276
65. Seki T, Wakabayashi M, Nakagawa T et al. (1999) Percutaneous microwave coagulation therapy for patients with small hepatocellular carcinoma: comparison with percutaneous ethanol injection therapy. Cancer 85:1694–1702
66. Shibata T, Niinobu T, Ogata N, Takami M (2000) Microwave coagulation therapy for multiple hepatic metastases from colorectal carcinoma. Cancer 89:276–284
67. Shibata T, Iimuro Y, Yamamoto Y et al. (2002) Small hepatocellular carcinoma: comparison of radio-frequency ablation and percutaneous microwave coagulation therapy. Radiology 223:331–337
68. Shiina S, Tagawa K, Unuma T et al. (1991) Percutaneous ethanol injection therapy for hepatocellular carcinoma: a histopathologic study. Cancer 68:1524–1530
69. Shiina S, Tagawa K, Niwa Y et al. (1993) Percutaneous ethanol injection therapy for hepatocellular carcinoma: results in 146 patients. AJR Am J Roentgenol 160:1023–1028
70. Solbiati L, Goldberg SN, Ierace T et al. (1997) Hepatic metastases: percutaneous radio-frequency ablation with cooled-tip electrodes. Radiology 205:367–373
71. Solbiati L, Livraghi T, Goldberg SN et al. (2001) Percutaneous radio-frequency ablation of hepatic metastases from colorectal cancer: long-term results in 117 patients. Radiology 221:159–166
72. Tateishi R, Shiina S, Teratani T et al. (2005) Percutaneous radiofrequency ablation for hepatocellular carcinoma. Cancer 103:1201–1209
73. Teratani T, Ishikawa T, Shiratori Y et al. (2002) Hepatocellular carcinoma in elderly patients: beneficial therapeutic efficacy using percutaneous ethanol injection therapy. Cancer 95:816–823
74. Vogl TJ, Muller PK, Hammerstingl R et al. (1995) Malignant liver tumors treated with MR imaging-guided laser-induced thermotherapy: technique and prospective results. Radiology 196:257–265
75. Vogl TJ, Straub R, Eichler K et al. (2002) Malignant liver tumors treated with MR imaging-guided laser-induced thermotherapy: experience with complications in 899 patients (2,520 lesions). Radiology 225:367–377
76. Vogl TJ, Straub R, Eichler K et al. (2004) Colorectal carcinoma metastases in liver: laser-induced interstitial thermotherapy – local tumor control rate and survival data. Radiology 230:450–458

77. Weitz J, Blumgart LH, Fong Y et al. (2005) Partial hepatectomy for metastases from noncolorectal, nonneuroendocrine carcinoma. Ann Surg 241:269–276
78. Wong LL, Tanaka K, Lau L, Komura S (2004) Pretransplant treatment of hepatocellular carcinoma: assessment of tumor necrosis in explanted livers. Clin Transplant 18:227–234
79. Wood TF, Rose DM, Chung M et al. (2000) Radiofrequency ablation of 231 unresectable hepatic tumors: indications, limitations, and complications. Ann Surg Oncol 7:593–600
80. Yamamoto J, Okada S, Shimada K et al. (2001) Treatment strategy for small hepatocellular carcinoma: comparison of long-term results after percutaneous ethanol injection therapy and surgical resection. Hepatology 34:707–713
81. Yamasaki T, Kurokawa F, Shirahashi H et al. (2002) Percutaneous radiofrequency ablation therapy for patients with hepatocellular carcinoma during occlusion of hepatic blood flow. Comparison with standard percutaneous radiofrequency ablation therapy. Cancer 95:2353–2360
82. Yamashiki N, Kato T, Bejarano PA et al. (2003) Histopathological changes after microwave coagulation therapy for patients with hepatocellular carcinoma: review of 15 explanted livers. Am J Gastroenterol 98:2052–2059

8 Lung Tumors

K. Steinke

8.1 Introduction

Lung cancer is the leading cause of cancer deaths in both men and women, causing more deaths than breast, prostate, and colorectal cancer combined. Eighty percent are non-small-cell lung cancer (NSCLC) and less than 20% of these patients can have a curative resection [1]. Pulmonary metastases are identified in up to 40% of patients dying of malignant tumors and can represent the only site of distant disease [2].

Resection of non-small-cell primary lung cancer and metastases from several extrapulmonary primary tumors (e.g., colorectal cancer, endocrine tumors, renal cell carcinoma, leiomyosarcoma, ENT tumors) has been shown to be much more effective in terms of survival than medical treatment alone [3].

Open thoracic surgery is a major invasive procedure performed under general anesthesia and associated with considerable morbidity and need for inpatient care [4].

8.2 Local Tumor Destruction

Methods for the local ablation modalities include the application of heat (radiofrequency ablation [RFA], laser-induced thermotherapy [LITT], microwave coagulation, and high-intensity focused ultrasound [HIFU]), cold (cryotherapy), ionizing irradiation (external, internal), photodynamic therapy, and electrochemotherapy. Some methods such as RFA and LITT within the hyperthermia modalities have been used more extensively than the other methods listed. Radiofrequency ablation is an evolving minimally invasive procedure for local control of unresectable primary and secondary pulmonary tumors [5–7]. The approach is percutaneous, under CT guidance.

8.3 Indications for Lung Radiofrequency Ablation

The indications for local destruction of lung tumor are similar to those established for resection, although with some modifications. It is usually felt that the number of lesions per hemithorax should not be more than six and that the largest lesion diameter should be less than 5 cm. Most authors think that the treatment should be offered only to patients with no evident extrapulmonary disease. Ideally tumors should be smaller than 3.5 cm in diameter and completely surrounded by nontumorous lung. Tumors abutting the pleura can be treated efficiently, but this is associated with increased pain during and after treatment.

The surgical trauma may contribute to recurrence, growth of metastases, and metastatic spread. These unwanted consequences of surgery depend on factors such as immunosuppression [8], shedding of tumor cells into the wounded area, and the circulation [9] and the production and release of growth factors for wound healing, which influence tumor cell adhesion and growth [10]. The potential advantages of local tumor destruction methods might include selective damage which leads to less immunosuppression and release of less growth factor, minimal treatment morbidity and mortality, less breathing impairment in patients with borderline lung function by sparing healthy lung tissue, repeatability, fairly low costs, excellent imaging during the procedure and for follow-up, and finally the gain in quality of life with less pain, much shorter hospitalization times, with the interventions performed on an outpatient basis or with overnight stays.

Following hyperthermic treatment, there are a number of events inducing favorable immunological effects, such as heat shock protein expression (HSP) within tumors [11], increased expression of cancer antigens [12], and increased lymphocyte adhesion to endothelial cells [13].

8.4 Technique of Radiofrequency Ablation of Lung Tumors

Five RF devices are currently available (Fig. 8.1a–e). The systems from RITA Medical Systems (Mountain View, CA, USA) (a) and Radiotherapeutics (Boston Scientific) (b) use deployable tines that expand into the tumor after an outer trocar is positioned at the tumor edge or in the tumor.

The Radionics device has different sizes of active (uninsulated) tips to create different ablation sizes. The system requires a pump that perfuses chilled saline through the hollow ports inside the needle in a closed system. The BERCHTOLD system infuses normal saline to increase the ablation area. The Celon-device (Celon AG, Tetlow, Germany) (e) is so far the only bipolar needle available.

Each monopolar device consists of an electrical generator, needle electrode, and grounding pad(s). The systems vary in the amount of generator power (50–250 W), generator cost (US $12 000–$30 000), use of electrode chilling, size and configuration of electrodes, electrode cost (US $500–$1800), use of infusion, infusion media, parameters monitored, algorithm used, and the amount of operator input. All electrodes are currently nonreusable.

8.5 Imaging and Real-Time Monitoring

In contrast to solid organs, lung parenchyma is not visible on ultrasound. Computed tomography (CT) and positron emission tomography (PET) for preoperative imaging, CT and magnetic resonance imaging (MRI) for intraoperative monitoring, and CT, PET, and MRI for follow-up are the imaging techniques in use. Although CT is not ideal for real-time monitoring because definitive thermal tissue changes are not visible within 24 h, a reproducible ovoid pulmonary opacification (ground-glass attenuation) can bee seen around the adequately ablated lesion, which is equivalent to the heat-damaged area and is sharply demarcated from the surrounding healthy tissue. Accordingly, technical success can be defined as the emergence of the surrounding ground-glass attenuation on a CT scan immediately after RF ablation [14].

MRI appears to be the ideal tool for temperature mapping. A particular advantage of MRI for guiding thermal procedures is that it not only allows temperature mapping but can be used as well for target definition, and it may provide an early evaluation of therapeutic efficacy [15]. However, availability is low and costs are high.

Fluorine 18 fluorodeoxyglucose (FDG), an analog of glucose, accumulates in most tumors in a greater amount than it does in normal tissue. FDG PET is being used in diagnosis and follow-up of several malignancies, lung cancer above all [16]. CT scanners are now being combined with PET scanners. The combined PET/CT devices offer several potential advantages over the PET scanner alone: better quality PET images because of the more accurate correction for attenuation provided by CT, automatic registration of CT (anatomic) and PET (metabolic) information, and shorter imaging times.

8.6 Procedure

Patients are selected in a joint tumor board. Patients amenable for RFA treatment are judged not suitable for surgery because of the site and distribution of their lung tumors or because of their limited cardiorespiratory function. Occa-

8 Lung Tumors

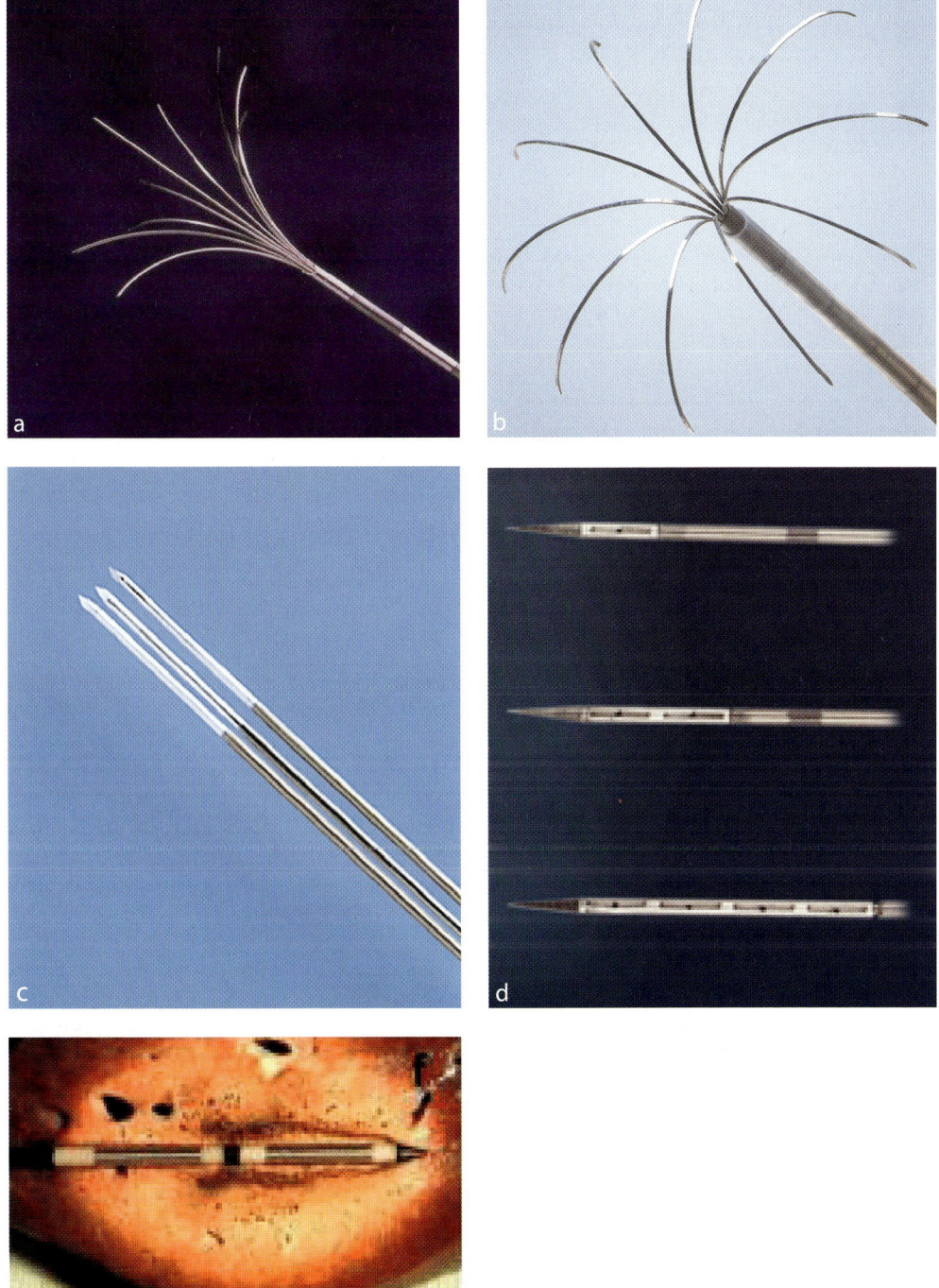

Fig. 8.1a–e Current devices for RFA of lung tumors

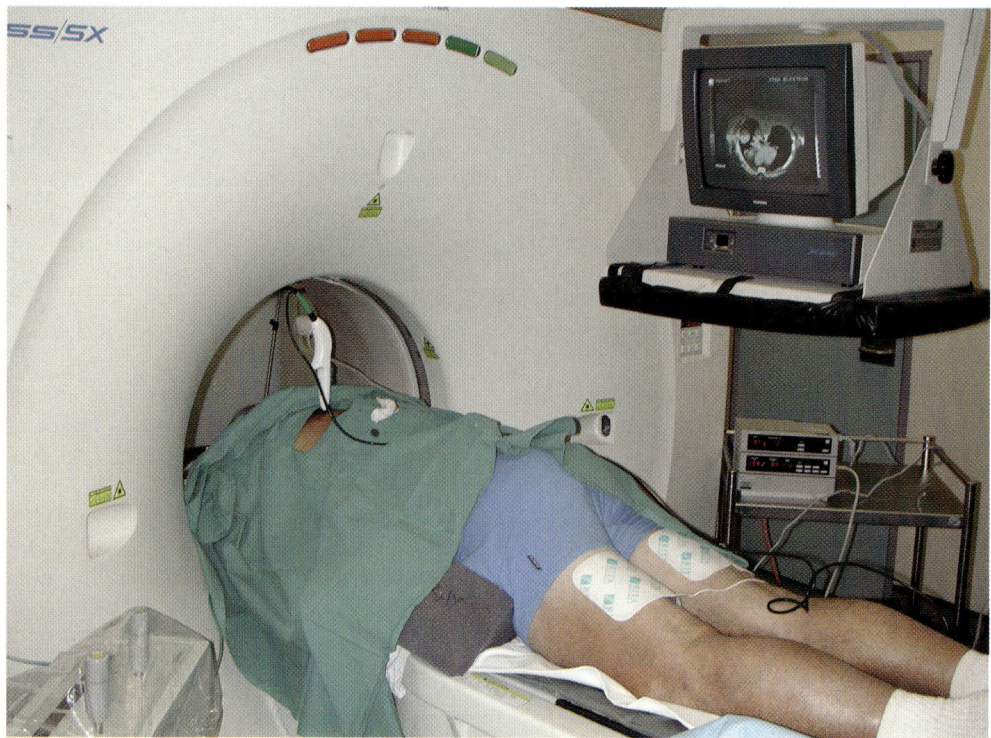

Fig. 8.2 CT suite with ongoing lung RFA

sional refusal of the patient to undergo major surgery despite qualification for it, opting for the less invasive alternative, does occur.

Bilateral metastases are treated, but for safety reasons only one lung at a time should be ablated.

In lesions greater than 3 cm in largest diameter overlapping ablations are required. Our exclusion criteria were and are an uncorrectable coagulopathy and more than six metastases per hemithorax.

The patient's informed consent is mandatory. The data reported in this chapter refers to radiofrequency ablations with the monopolar deployable RITA StarBurst XL electrode, which creates ablations up to 5 cm in diameter. This device has nine active electrodes (five with thermocouples), and an active trocar tip. Electrodes are well distributed, for a "space-filling" globe design, with one electrode straight along the axis of the probe, four curved electrodes around the "equator" and the remaining four curved electrodes along the "northern hemisphere" [5]. The thermocouples are located in the tip of the straight electrode plus in four of the electrodes around the equator. These thermocouples are used to provide temperature feedback for monitoring, ablation control and tissue temperature after ablation.

Data from the generator (power, impedance, temperature, time, etc.) can be collected and graphically displayed on a computer.

Patients are provided with an intravenous access. The patient is positioned on the CT table according to the location of the lesion(s) (Fig.8.2). Mindful that the ablation procedure takes at least 15 min per lesion at target temperature, the patient should be positioned as comfortably as possible, preferably supine or prone. Patient blood pressure, pulse rate, and blood oxygen saturation via a pulse oximeter are monitored and recorded.

To lessen the risk of skin burns, the grounding pads should be positioned far away from the thorax. When procedures where a large amount of RF energy is delivered to the patient, repeated checking of the grounding pad temperature is advisable to avoid skin burns.

The intervention is performed under sterile conditions with the patient draped and prepped as usual.

The tissue down to the pleura is anesthetized with local anesthetic. Sedation/analgesia generally consists of conscious sedation – usually the combination of sedatives and analgetics the department is familiar with – that can be given and increased on demand.

Publications on liver RFA and the data from a world survey on lung RFA advocate analgosedation as the sedation of choice in the routine setting. We use conscious sedation, managed by a qualified nurse with radiologist supervision with no adverse event to date. Very occasional agitation despite (or due to) profound sedation is sometimes observed, usually not requiring any special intervention. Not having to depend on anesthetic service allows greater flexibility in RF procedures/CT room management and is cost-effective. We presume that general anesthesia could be necessary in procedures that are long or painful, with either broad pleural contact of the tumor or where the patient is likely to be agitated or to move. Prophylactic intravenous antibiotics should be administered.

Because of the CT gantry limiting space, it is possible to use only 10-cm and 15-cm probes, with the 25-cm probes mostly used for laparoscopic treatments. The electrode is positioned under CT guidance; CT fluoroscopy is preferred. Guidance without fluoroscopy is more complicated and thus less precise due to the breathing-related motion. With CT fluoroscopy, the radiation exposure for the patient is decreased because the electrodes are placed in the tumor more quickly with real-time visual control [17]. Clinicians performing the procedure can minimize their radiation exposure by using a tool such as an artery clamp to grasp and move the device during scanning.

Similar to diagnostic biopsies, the radiologist should chose the access site least likely to damage vessels or nerves, minimizing pleural crossing and allowing for a minimum depth of the electrode inside the thoracic cage to reduce displacement due to breathing, motion, or generator cable weight.

Once the needle tip is in the right place, the tines are deployed to a 2-cm array and the probe is connected to the generator. One should be alert of the risk of "push back," in that instead of forwarding the electrodes from the device's trocar and into the tumor, the trocar is pushed backward, exposing the electrodes proximal to the tumor and not penetrating the tumor, as intended.

The protocol we use recommends a power setting at 50 W, adjustable to 200 W, and a temperature setting at 90 °C. The aim is a gradual heating leading to coagulation necrosis. We attempt to avoid charring with subsequent loss of heat dissipation by starting with a lower power setting. A thermal lesion of coagulation necrosis encompasses the tumor and a 5–10 mm surrounding safety margin of normal healthy tissue (Fig. 8.3a–e).

The ideal size of the lesion should be less than 3 cm in biggest diameter and thus treatable with a single ablation. The ideal shape of the lesion is spherical. In lesions larger than 3 cm, overlapping ablations are required.

Intermittent radiological confirmation of the position of the probe should be performed, especially after changing deployment size or if the patient has moved significantly. When the average temperature has been maintained for the required duration, the generator automatically switches off. The electrodes are retracted into the trocar. To reduce the risk of tumor seeding and lessen the risk of hemorrhage while retracting the probe, track ablation is performed by turning down the output, while drawing the needle out slowly to thoroughly coagulate the tissue around the track.

8.7 Patient Follow-Up

Depending on the depth of analgosedation, the patient should be monitored up to 4 h after the procedure and continuously monitored for pulse, blood pressure, and blood oxygen saturation. An erect chest X-ray 4 h after the procedure and another one before discharge should be routinely performed and assessed for pneumothorax and

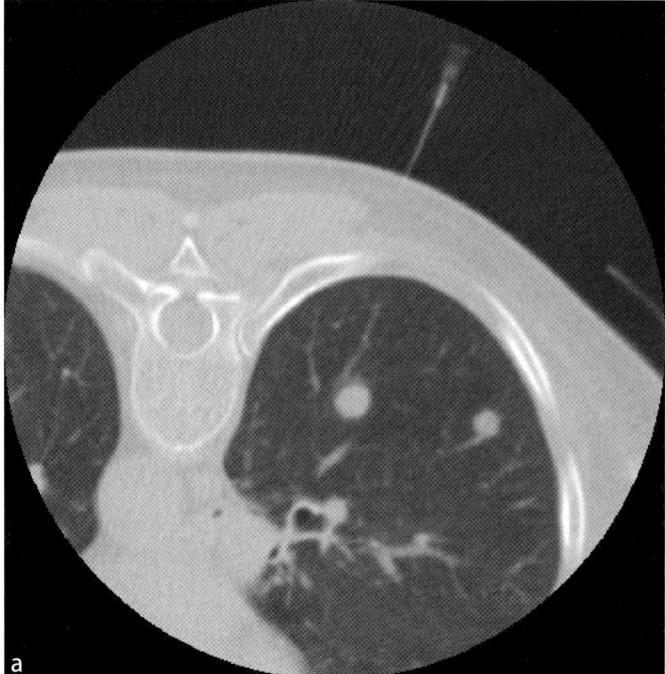

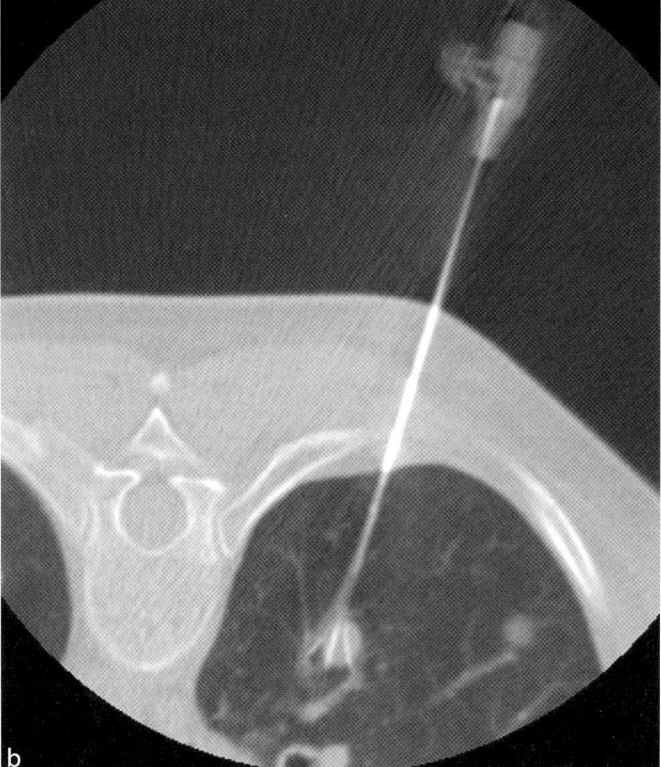

Fig. 8.3 **a** Axial CT prone position, lung window. Two metastases in the right lower lobe (RLL). **b** Start of RFA of medial metastasis; **c** end of RFA medial metastasis, ovoid opacification surrounding the active needle region, consistent with ablation area; **d** cavitation of ablation area; **e** end of RFA session with demarcation of both ablation areas

8 Lung Tumors

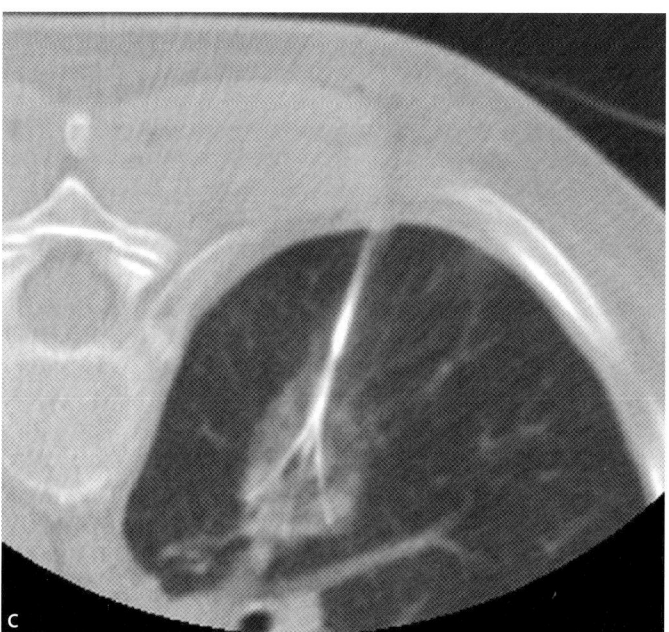

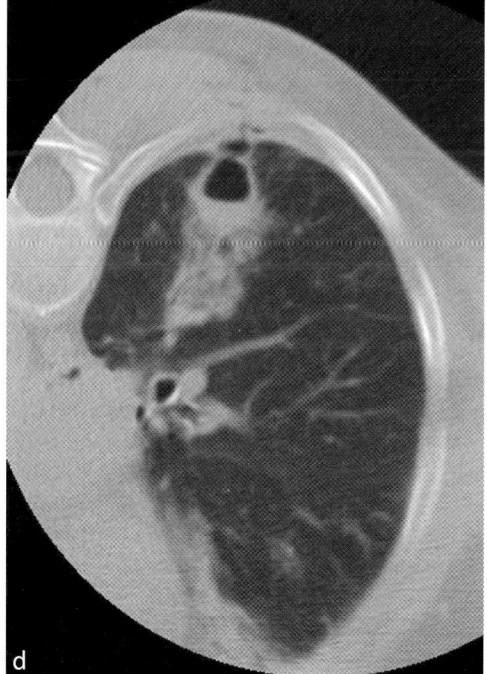
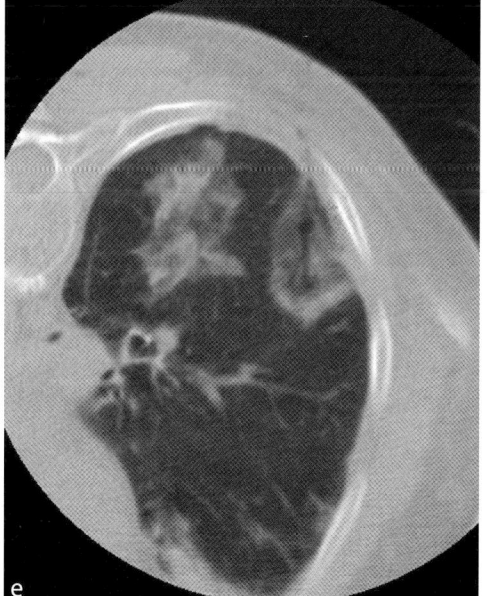

pleural effusion. A hemorrhage not visible during the procedure is very unlikely to occur thereafter.

Chest CT follow-ups at 1 month, then at 3-month intervals after ablation within the 1st year followed by 6-month intervals thereafter is one of the common follow-up schemes.

The size of the ablated lesions and their contrast uptake is assessed. In technically successful ablations, our experience has shown an initial increase in size compared to the pretreatment lesion, as the ablation area not only encompasses the lesion, but also a surrounding safety margin. This is followed by a gradual involution of the ablation area [18]. Residual scars are the rule and they are usually permanent (Fig. 8.4).

The 1-month follow-up CT scan measurement is obtained as a post-RF reference measurement with any further increase in size or in attenuation suspicious of recurrence.

PET is also a very good and sensitive procedure for follow-up [19] of ablated primary lung cancer and many tumors of metastatic origin [20], providing a better discrimination between residual granulation tissue and recurrent tumor.

can be inserted into the sedated patient. Upon re-expansion of the lung, the ablation can still be successfully continued.

A major problem is desiccated tissue that adheres to the electrode and forms an electrically insulating coating, resulting in charring, which can prevent the easy withdrawal of the electrodes into the trocar (Fig. 8.7).

Charring can prevent the intended dissipation of the heat away from the electrodes, resulting in a sudden rise in the measured system impedance (above 500 ohms) and a corresponding decrease in the delivered power. This can result in the generator automatically switching off [21]. Pausing the RF for 30–60 s to allow conductive body fluids to rehydrate the tissue or retracting and redeploying the electrodes to "clean" the adherent charred tissue from the electrodes may allow an electrical connection to be reestablished. Forceful withdrawal of the device could cause tissue injury along the probe track [22].

After the procedure, most patients experience some pain, usually pleuritic in type, which is typically treated with nonopioid analgesics. Al-

8.8 Complications

The combination of a hard tumor in soft lung sometimes can make tumor penetration difficult. If a hard tumor bounces away from the electrode, it is advisable to attempt to deploy the tines by 2–3 mm and then spike the lesion with the leading tip of the straight electrode (Fig. 8.5) before a further approach at transfixing the tumor from another access site.

Repositioning and multiple attempts to transfix the tumor are likely to lead to hemorrhage and moderately large pneumothoraces (Fig. 8.6). Should a pneumothorax occur with subsequent retraction of the targeted lesion, a chest drain

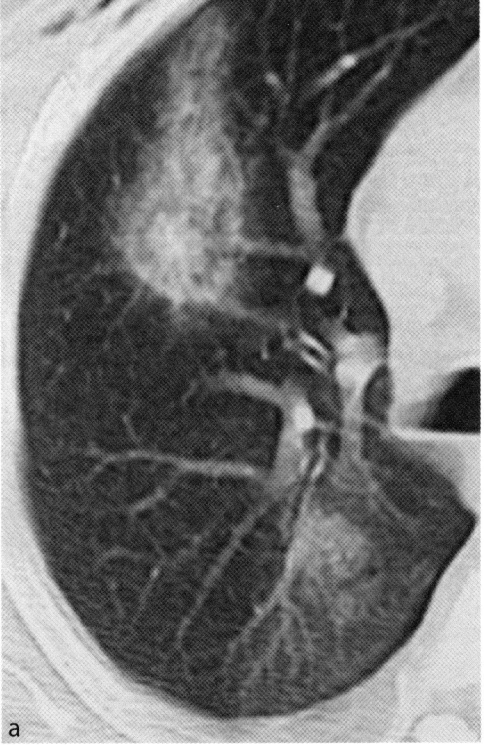

Fig. 8.4 a Post-RFA of 1.2-cm metastasis in the right upper lobe (RUL) with ovoid opacification around the probe; **b** 1 week after RFA with opacification measuring 3.0 × 3.5 cm; **c** 3 months after RFA, opacification measuring 1.5 × 1.5 cm, but less dense than before; **d** 6 months after RFA, opacification measuring 1.4 × 1.3 cm, opacification size unchanged but looking shrunken; **e** 12 months after RFA, residual scar

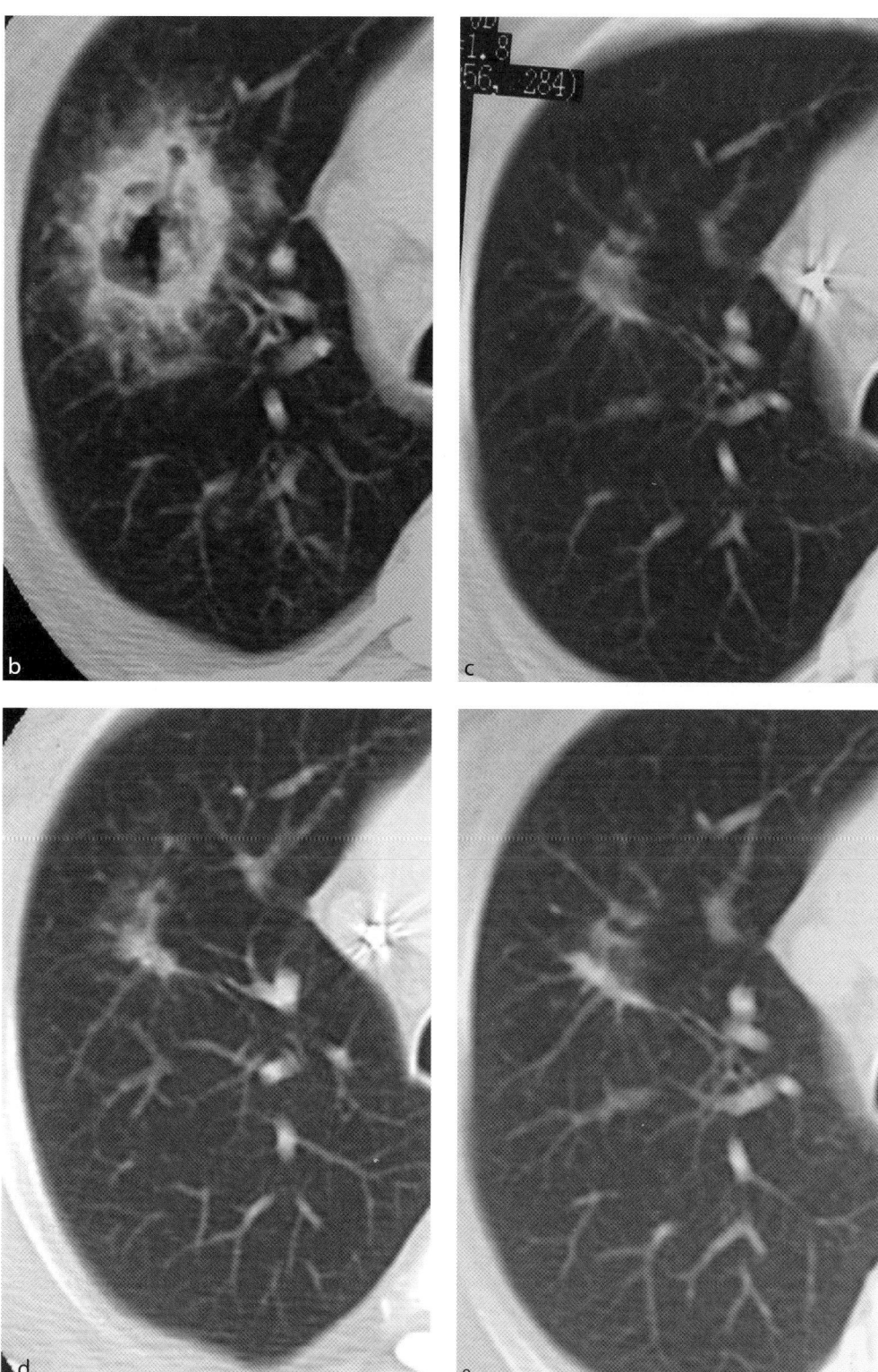

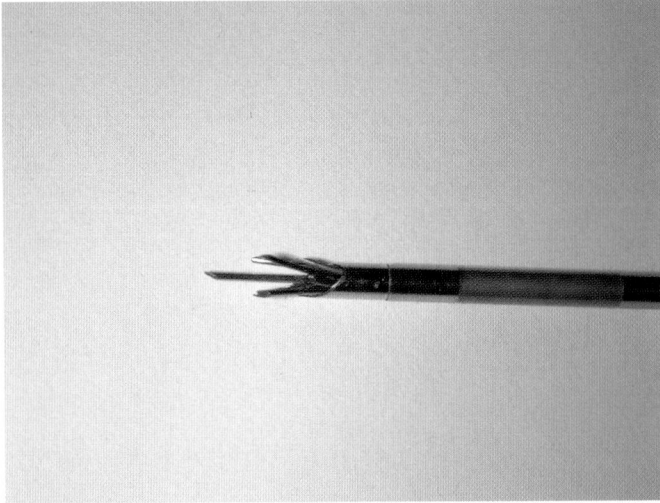

Fig. 8.5 Slightly deployed tines with thin central electrode along probe axis

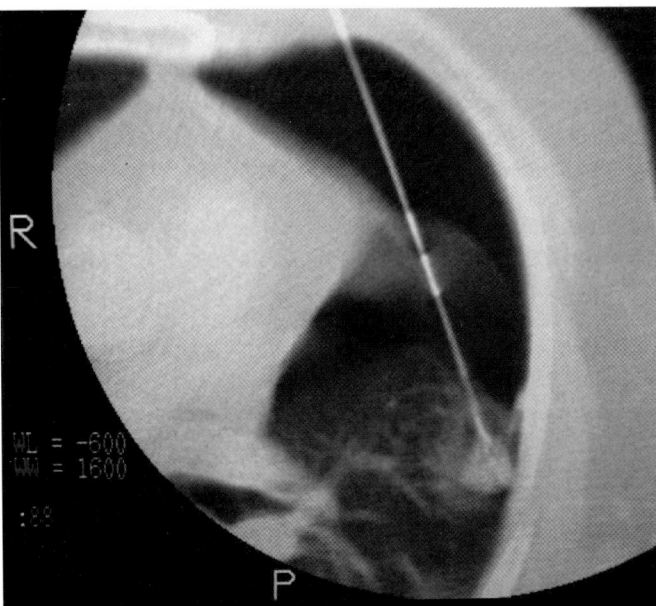

Fig. 8.6 Large basal pneumothorax at RFA, increased during ablation procedure

though less than 5% of patients require stronger pain medication, it is advisable to be liberal with analgesia, allowing deep respiration and preventing possible superinfection of the treated, suboptimally aerated lung portion. Fever, with slightly raised temperatures (< 39 °C) is often observed in patients for up to 1 week after ablation. Patients may also develop pneumonia/abscess formation, but there usually will be symptoms in addition to the raised temperature, such as chills and severe coughing.

Sympathetic pleural effusion to an amount that does not require tapping is often seen on the upright postablation chest X-ray with obliteration of the ipsilateral posterior and lateral costophrenic angle. Symptomatic effusions requiring tapping occur in less than 5% of the procedures, usually after multiple ablations, and are often hemorrhagic.

Pneumothorax occurs fairly commonly, approximately one-third of the patients with metastatic lung disease of extrapulmonary origin

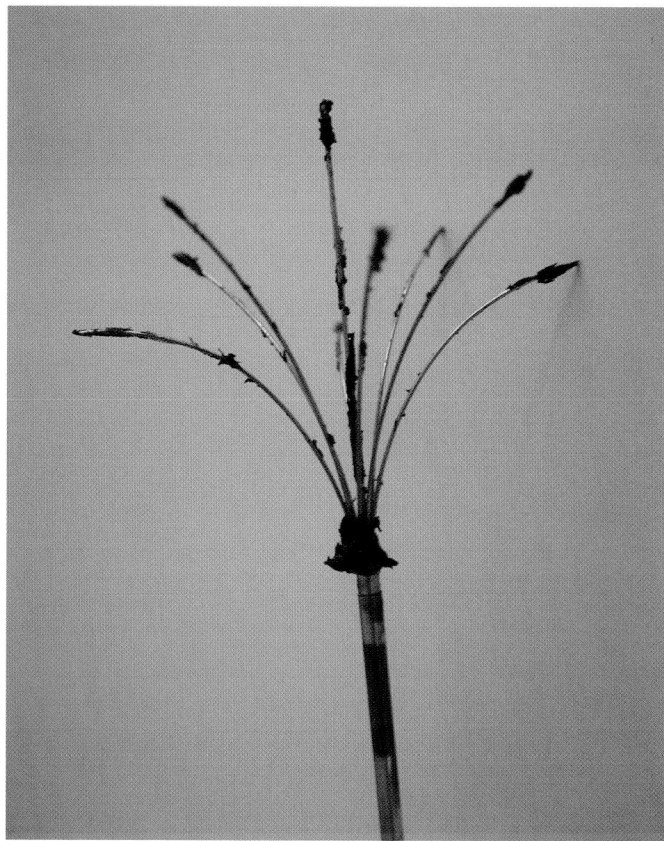

Fig. 8.7 Charred lung tissue sticking to the electrodes

and half of the patients with primary lung cancer (not abutting the pleural surface) develop a pneumothorax during the ablation procedure. Pneumothorax occurs more often with multiple procedures. According to our data in patients who developed a pneumothorax, an average of 2.6 lesions were treated compared with 1.4 lesions treated in those without pneumothorax [18]. Roughly one-third of the pneumothoraces require chest tubes.

Cavitation within the ablated area is a frequent observation within the 1st week after ablation, seen in one-fifth of the tumors treated, frequently seen when the size of the lesion at 1 week after treatment exceeds the size of the pretreatment lesion by 200% or more [18]. Cavitations usually resolve spontaneously over the first few weeks, occasional access to adjacent bronchi with coughing up of desiccated tissue and superinfection with abscess formation does occur (Fig. 8.8a–c).

Hemorrhage is a known complication in lung RFA, and results from the positioning of the device, as seen in lung biopsies, rather than from the ablative procedure. Intraparenchymal hemorrhage is usually mild, self-limiting, and of little clinical significance, but it is a complication to be aware of. The more centrally the lesion is located and the larger the adjacent vessels are, the higher the likelihood of a substantial hemorrhage. Despite a hemorrhage – provided the patient shows no signs of distress – it is advisable to continue the ablative procedure if the tumor has not been masked by the hemorrhage, as the ablative heat often cauterizes the leaking vessel.

Severe second- and third-degree burns (Fig. 8.9) at the grounding pad site have been reported, both after open liver RFA and after percutaneous liver RFA [23]. All dispersive pads were believed to having been placed correctly; at the end of the ablation procedures, none of the pads had been noticed as having been improperly at-

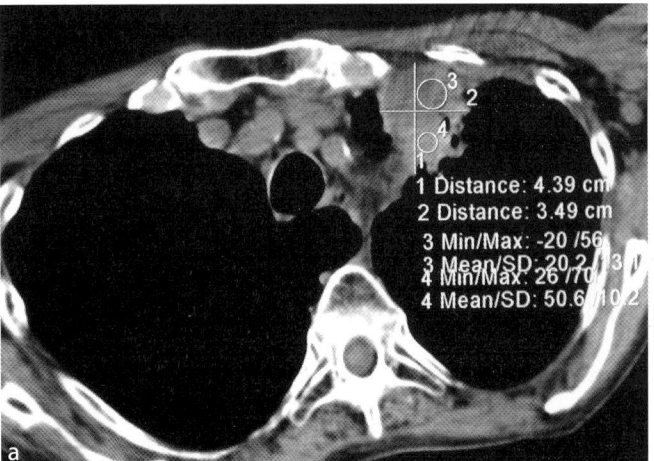
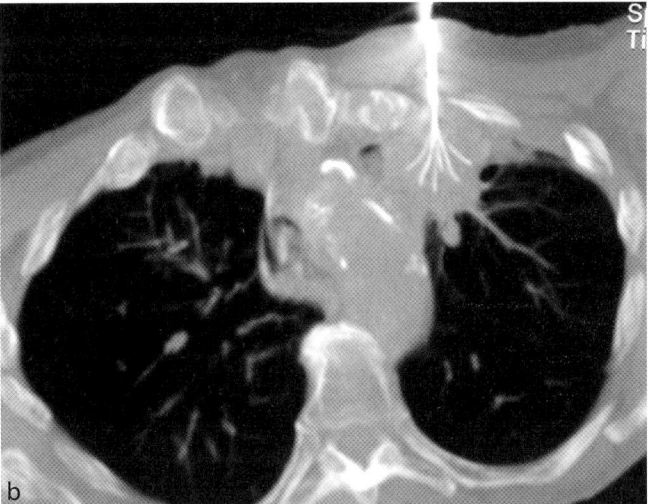
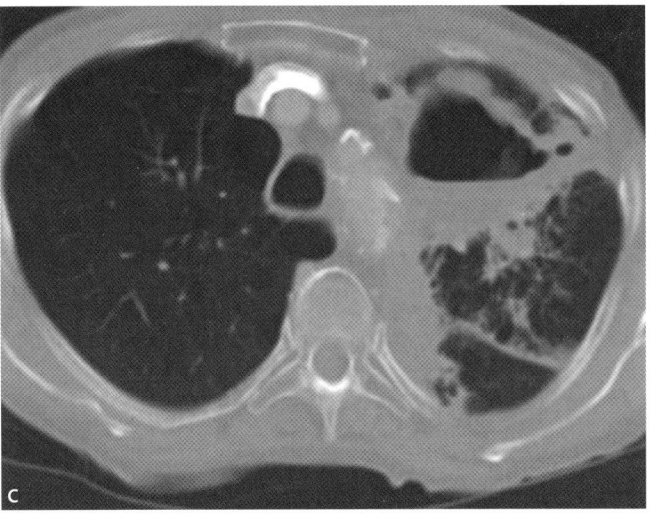

Fig. 8.8 a Paramediastinal NSCLC in the left upper lobe (LUL); b RFA; c large abscess within ablation area 1 month after ablation

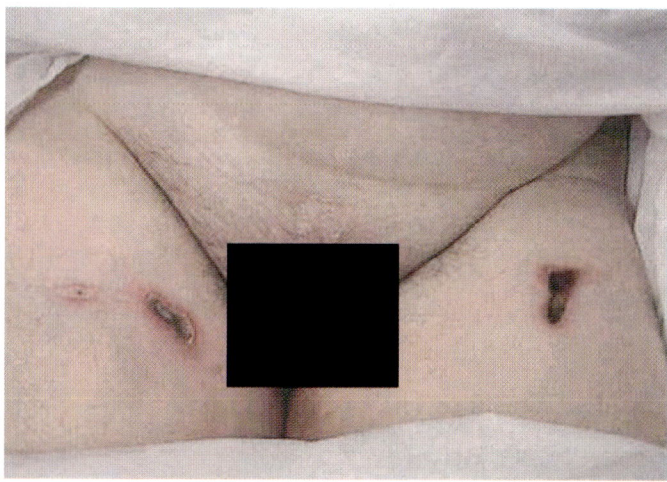

Fig. 8.9 Third-degree skin burns at the grounding pad site on both thighs seen 1 week after a prolonged RFA session

tached to the skin. In our opinion and according to our experience, the complication of pad burns seems to be underestimated, in particular the rate of mild skin irritations seems to get lost to the follow-up, as patients are usually discharged the same day or the day after the (percutaneous) procedure, and they probably do not consider it worth mentioning.

The orientation of the dispersive pads was shown by Goldberg et al. to be an important factor in the maximum temperature that is reached in the skin at the pad site [24]. The leading edge is the site of maximum power concentration and therefore the side of the pad with the largest edge should face the active electrode. Skin preparation with shaving of the area the pads are to be placed on and properly cleaning the skin are essential to avoid poor contact. The position of the single pad, as in diathermy, is not very important except to say that it should not be placed over bony prominence or scars. The placement of multiple pads requires greater attention in that the level and the distance of the pads relative to each other and to the active electrode should be similar to avoid the current returning through the closest pad and therefore resulting in overly high current density and burns.

8.9 Clinical Outcome

Surgical resection of lung metastases is an established therapy for a large number of primary tumors, but there is some controversy about prognostic factors for long-term survival. The long-term results and prognostic analysis based on 5206 cases of the International Registry of Lung Metastases showed that complete resection is the principal prognostic index with an actuarial survival after complete metastasectomy of 36% at 5 years, 26% at 10 years and 22% at 15 years [25]. Lung cancer is the commonest cause of cancer death in both sexes worldwide, with most often advanced and incurable disease at time of diagnosis. Based on current projected smoking patterns, it is anticipated that lung cancer will remain the leading cause of cancer death in the world for the coming decades.

In primary lung cancer less than one-fifth of the patients are amenable for curative resection. A considerable proportion of these patients suffers from cardiopulmonary co-morbidities, which constitute a significant risk both for the surgery itself and for the recovery period due to critical residual lung volume to maintain proper function. Since 1999/2000, well over 1000 patients worldwide have been radiofrequency ablated for their lung tumors. There is no published data available on prognostic factors for lung RFA, partly because this treatment modality is very new and there are not sufficiently long follow-up periods to date, partly because of the inhomogeneous inclusion criteria, different ablation devices, different ablation protocols, and the lack of standardization of terminology and reporting criteria [26].

The type of resection does not seem to significantly affect survival according to a study on 85 patients who underwent pulmonary metastasectomy by either conventional resections with diathermy dissection or stapler suture lines, lobectomy or laser ablation with an Nd:YAG laser [27].

Even sequential metastasectomies seem to have a favorable outcome. Multiple attempts to reestablish intrathoracic control of metastatic disease seems to be justified in carefully selected patients, but the magnitude of benefit is reported to decline with each subsequent attempt [28].

Lung RFA has been so far mainly applied to unresectable tumors and mostly in a palliative approach. Outcomes therefore cannot be compared to surgery, as there is a significant bias in patient inclusion criteria and thus in life expectancy. Prospective randomized trials are not available. Histological proof of completeness of tissue heat destruction through percutaneous lung RFA has been given [29] and confirmed by several short-term follow-up studies [30–32].

Current data suggest that RFA is most suitable for tumors less than 4 cm in largest diameter and is better for peripheral rather than centrally based nodules. Additionally, studies of RFA followed by resection have demonstrated a learning-curve effect with improved tumor kill in the later cases performed in these series [33].

It cannot yet be claimed that percutaneous RFA will have equivalent results to resection. The aim of this treatment modality is, however, to achieve complete local tumor ablation without the additional factors and complications inherent with a surgical procedure: general anesthesia, chest tube drainage, longer hospital stay, and substantial loss of healthy pulmonary tissue.

Radiofrequency ablation is a good option for those patients who are believed to be at increased risk for resection or who refuse resection, when operation would otherwise be the appropriate therapy.

The evaluation of standardized quality-of-life questionnaires for lung RFA showed that the procedure is associated with a minor decrease in quality of life at 1 month, which had returned to baseline at 3 months [34].

8.10 Outlook

If long-term results should parallel those of liver RFA treatment, lung RFA might also be a new alternative to lung surgery or radiation. The well-established data on survival after pulmonary surgery makes us confident enough to state that if we are able to completely ablate lung tumors by RFA we can achieve comparable survival rates to surgical tumor removal. Lower morbidity and mortality, as well as a better quality of life accompany this treatment, with the possibility of treating patients on an overnight or even outpatient base.

Bipolar electrodes currently under development will enable faster and safer ablations. Additionally, RFA can be used for local control of peripheral tumors in patients with more advanced cancers in combination with other therapies, such as radiation or chemotherapy.

References

1. Brescia FJ (2001) Lung cancer – a philosophical, ethical, and personal perspective. Crit Rev Oncol Hematol 40:139–148
2. Davidson RS, Nwogu CE, Brentjens MJ, Anderson TM (2001) The surgical management of pulmonary metastasis: current concepts. Surg Oncol 10:35–42
3. Landreneau RJ, Sugarbaker DJ, Mack MJ et al. (1997) Wedge resection versus lobectomy for stage I (T1 N0 M0) non-small-cell lung cancer. J Thorac Cardiovasc Surg 113:691–698
4. Ferguson MK, Durkin AE (2003) A comparison of three scoring systems for predicting complications after major lung resection. Eur J Cardiothorac Surg 23:35–42
5. Rossi S, Di Stasi M, Buscarini E et al. (1996) Percutaneous RF interstitial thermal ablation in the treatment of hepatic cancer. AJR 16:759–768
6. Berber E, Flesher NL, Siperstein AE (2000) Initial clinical evaluation of the RITA 5-centimeter radiofrequency thermal ablation catheter in the treatment of liver tumors. Cancer J 6:319–329
7. Scudamore C (2000) Volumetric radiofrequency ablation: technical consideration. Cancer J 6:316–318

8. Colacchio TA, Yeager MP, Hildebrandt LW (1994) Perioperative immunomodulation in cancer surgery. Am J Surg 167:174–179
9. Hansen E, Wolff N, Knuechel R, Ruschoff J, Hofstaedter F, Taeger K (1995) Tumor cells in blood shed from the surgical field. Arch Surg 130:387–393
10. Brown LM, Malkinson AM, Rannels DE, Rannels SR (1999) Compensatory lung growth after partial pneumonectomy enhances lung tumorigenesis induced by 3-methylcholanthrene. Cancer Res 59:5089–5092
11. Srivastava P (2002) Roles of heat-shock proteins in innate and adaptive immunity. Nat Rev Immunol 2:185–194
12. Gromkowski SH, Yagi J, Janeway CA Jr (1989) Elevated temperature regulates tumor necrosis factor-mediated immune killing. Eur J Immunol 19:1709–1714
13. Lefor AT, Foster CE 3rd, Sartor W, Engbrecht B, Fabian DF, Silverman D (1994) Hyperthermia increases intercellular adhesion molecule-1 expression and lymphocyte adhesion to endothelial cells. Surgery 116:214–220
14. Yasui K, Kanazawa S, Sano Y, Fujiwara T, Kagawa S, Mimura H, Dendo S, Mukai T, Fujiwara H, Iguchi T, Hyodo T, Shimizu N, Tanaka N, Hiraki Y (2004) Thoracic tumors treated with CT-guided radiofrequency ablation: initial experience. Radiology 231:850–857
15. Quesson B, de Zwart JA, Moonen CT (2000) Magnetic resonance temperature imaging for guidance of thermotherapy. J Magn Reson Imaging 12:525–533
16. Rohren EM, Turkington TG, Coleman RE (2004) Clinical applications of PET in oncology. Radiology 231:305–332
17. Carlson SK, Bender CE, Classic KL, Zink FE, Quam JP, Ward EM, Oberg AL (2001) Benefits and safety of CT fluoroscopy in interventional radiologic procedures. Radiology 219:515–520
18. Steinke K, King J, Glenn D, Morris DL (2003) Radiologic appearance and complications of percutaneous computed tomography-guided radiofrequency-ablated pulmonary metastases from colorectal carcinoma. J Comput Assist Tomogr 27:750–757
19. MacManus MP, Hicks RJ, Matthews JP et al. (2003) Positron emission tomography is superior to computed tomography scanning for response-assessment after radical radiotherapy or chemoradiotherapy in patients with non-small-cell lung cancer. J Clin Oncol 21:1285–1292
20. Aquino SL (2005) Imaging of metastatic disease to the thorax. Radiol Clin North Am 43:481–495
21. Scudamore C (2000) Volumetric radiofrequency ablation: technical consideration. Cancer J 6:316–318
22. Steinke K, King J, Glenn D, Morris DL (2003) Percutaneous radiofrequency ablation of pulmonary metastases: difficulties withdrawing the hooks resulting in a split needle. Cardiovasc Intervent Radiol 26:583–585
23. Steinke K, Gananandha S, King J, Zhao J, Morris DL (2003) Dispersive pad site burns with modern radiofrequency ablation equipment. Surg Laparosc Endosc Percutan Tech 13:366–371
24. Goldberg SN, Solbiati L, Halpern EF, Gazelle GS (2000) Variables affecting proper system grounding for radiofrequency ablation in an animal model. JVIR 11:1069–1075
25. Friedel G, Pastorino U, Buyse M, Ginsberg RJ, Girard P, Goldstraw P, Johnston M, McCormack P, Pass H, Putnam JB, Toomes H (1999) Resection of lung metastases: long-term results and prognostic analysis based on 5206 cases – the International Registry of Lung Metastases. Zentralbl Chir 124:96–103
26. Goldberg SN, Grassi CJ, Cardella JF, Charboneau JW, Dodd GD 3rd, Dupuy DE, Gervais D, Gillams AR, Kane RA, Lee FT Jr, Livraghi T, McGahan J, Phillips DA, Rhim H, Silverman SG; Society of Interventional Radiology Technology Assessment Committee; International Working Group on Image-Guided Tumor Ablation (2005) Image-guided tumor ablation: standardization of terminology and reporting criteria. Radiology 235:728–739
27. Mineo TC, Ambrogi V, Tonini G, Nofroni I (2001) Pulmonary metastasectomy: might the type of resection affect survival? J Surg Oncol 76:47–52
28. Jaklitsch MT, Mery CM, Lukanich JM et al. (2001) Sequential thoracic metastasectomy prolongs survival by re-establishing local control within the chest. J Thorac Cardiovasc Surg 121:657–667

29. Steinke K, Habicht J, Thomsen S, Jacob LA (2002) CT-guided radiofrequency ablation of a pulmonary metastasis followed by surgical resection: a case report. Cardiovasc Intervent Radiol 25:543–546
30. Steinke K, Glenn D, King J, Clark W, Zhao J, Clingan P, Morris DL (2004) Percutaneous imaging-guided radiofrequency ablation (RFA) in patients with colorectal pulmonary metastases – 1-year follow-up. Ann Surg Oncol 11:207–212
31. Steinke K, Sewell P, Dupuy D, Lencioni R, Helmberger T, Kee ST, Jacob LA, King J, Glenn D, Morris DL (2004) Pulmonary radiofrequency ablation – an international study survey. Anticancer Res 24:339–344
32. Gadaleta C, Catino A, Ranieri G, Armenise F, Colucci G, Lorusso V, Cramarossa A, Fiorentini G, Mattioli V (2004) Radiofrequency thermal ablation of 69 lung neoplasms. J Chemother 16 [Suppl 5]:86–89
33. Fernando HC, Hoyos AD, Litle V, Belani CP, Luketich JD (2004) Radiofrequency ablation: identification of the ideal patient. Clin Lung Cancer 6:149–153
34. King J, Glenn D, Clark W, Zhao J, Steinke K, Clingan P, Morris DL (2004) Percutaneous imaging-guided radio frequency ablation of 45 pulmonary metastases in 20 patients with colorectal carcinoma. Br J Surg 91:217–223

9 Renal Tumors

Andreas Mahnken, Joseph Tacke

9.1 Introduction

During 2004, the American Cancer Society reported 35 710 new cases and estimated 12 480 deaths from renal cancer [1]. While historically renal cell carcinoma (RCC) was detected by flank pain and hematuria, the development of imaging techniques such as ultrasound (US) and computed tomography (CT) led to an increased detection rate of small renal tumors [2]. Further advances in cross-sectional imaging with introduction of multislice spiral CT (MSCT) and high-field magnetic resonance (MR) imaging in clinical routine and the more widespread availability of cross-sectional imaging have resulted in even earlier tumor detection. About two-thirds of all RCCs are now discovered incidentally [3]. However, the differentiation of small renal tumors remains difficult [4]. The natural history of renal tumors is variable but histological tumor type and tumor stage are important prognostic factors, with a survival advantage attributed to smaller tumors [5, 6]. Moreover, tumors less than 4 cm in diameter rarely metastasize.

The traditional treatment of RCC was open radical nephrectomy [7]. More frequent detection of small tumors pushed the development of less invasive operation techniques such as nephron-sparing partial nephrectomy via an open or laparoscopic approach. These techniques were successfully introduced into clinical routine [8]. The 10-year tumor-free survival rates were greater than 85% following nephron-sparing surgery [9, 10]. Initially limited to patients with bilateral disease or solitary kidney, nephron-sparing surgery is now also used for patients with healthy contralateral kidney [11]. These convincing results equal nephrectomy and pushed the development of new therapeutic concepts and the introduction of even less invasive, energy-based treatment options. Several of these thermal ablation techniques are now subject to clinical investigation, including radiofrequency (RF) ablation, cryotherapy, laser-induced thermotherapy (LITT), microwave ablation, and high-intensity focused ultrasound. Especially image-guided percutaneous radiofrequency ablation (RFA) has gained increasing attention as a minimally invasive treatment option for focal destruction of solid tumors. This technique provides several advantages over surgical resection, including reduced morbidity and the ability to treat poor surgical candidates. Moreover, in some patients it can be used as an outpatient therapy.

So far, the greatest attention has been given to RFA for the treatment of colorectal metastases to the liver and hepatocellular carcinoma. More recently, however, the clinical potential of RFA has greatly expanded. In particular, the kidney showed significant growth as a target for RFA. Impelling factors include the improved detection of RCC and the more extensive availability of RF systems. These factors led many investigators to assess the feasibility and efficacy of RFA for renal tumors. First used in 1997 [12], renal RFA has become an established treatment modality.

9.2 Experimental Investigations

Several animal studies have been directed toward determining the immediate or short-term histopathologic changes following RFA of normal porcine kidneys or of VX2 tumors implanted in rabbit kidneys. The animal's kidney demonstrated the zone of RFA as a sharply delineated area [13, 14]. On early microscopy, increased cytoplasmic eosinophilia, loss of cell border integrity, blurring of nuclear chromatin, and interstitial hemorrhage are visible. By day 3, typical coagulative necrosis develops. Inflammatory and fibroblastic changes occur between ablated kidney and the adjacent healthy renal parenchyma. Nuclear degeneration is complete by day 14 and necrosis is complete without features of renal parenchyma by day 30. From the center to the periphery, five different zones are described from histology: complete necrosis, inflammatory infiltrate, hemorrhage, fibrosis, and regeneration [15]. In rabbits, the renal medulla has been more sensitive to RFA than the renal cortex [16]. This is thought to result from the increased ion concentration in the medulla with augmentation of frictional energy and heating.

As induction of necrosis with RFA requires a temperature above 60 °C, well-perfused tissue such as the renal parenchyma may limit the size of the necrosis due to a heat sink. This potential disadvantage of RFA is caused by the cooling effect from the blood flow. Thus the effects of temporary renal ischemia have been evaluated in an animal model aiming at an increase of the lesion size. Immediate postmortem analysis after transfemoral balloon occlusion of the renal artery as well as selective embolization using particles led to a significant increase in lesion size in the ischemic kidney [17, 18]. Another study with laparoscopic renal hilar occlusion showed larger lesion sizes in the ischemic kidneys than the nonischemic kidneys 2 and 4 weeks after ablation, but the lesion sizes were not significantly different at 4 weeks [19]. Nevertheless, these results illustrate the ability to modify the size of necrosis by modulation of the renal perfusion.

9.3   Indication and Technique

So far there is no substantial long-term follow-up data available on renal RFA. Therefore, a comparison with the surgical reference standard of nephrectomy is not yet possible. Until then, renal RFA remains limited to selected patients. To provide all viable treatment options to a patient and to select the right patients for RFA, close collaboration between urologists, oncologist, and interventional radiologist is essential.

For patients with contraindications for surgery, especially co-morbid conditions or those patients who refuse open surgery, RFA is a promising treatment option. Further widely accepted indications include patients with a solitary kidney, multiple RCCs (Fig. 9.1), von Hippel Lindau disease, or limited renal function. Some centers limit treatment with curative intent to patients with greater than 1 year life expectancy [20]. A rare palliative indication is treatment of refractory hematuria [21]. Still, there are no uniform indications for renal RFA. In selected patients RFA may be considered an innovative therapy and even successful ablation of a Wilms tumor refractory to chemotherapy in a multimorbid child with a solitary kidney has been reported [22].

Many investigators limited the RFA to patients without metastatic disease. Some reports, however, indicate that isolated foci of metastatic disease can also be treated successfully with radiofrequency ablation [23, 24]. Further indications for RFA in RCC also include the palliative treatment of painful osseous metastases [25].

Several approaches have been reported to apply RF to the kidney. These include open surgical exposure, laparoscopic exposure, and an entirely percutaneous approach. Animal experiments showed no difference in the results using different approaches to the kidney [15]. In all techniques, hyperthermal effect on tumor tissue results in coagulation necrosis, which scars over time. In order to completely destroy the tumor, heat must exceed the tumor margin into healthy renal parenchyma. Although modern RF systems generate necrosis of 1.6–5 cm [26], most tumors need overlapping ablations, as the tumor geometry and the shape of the ablation zone often do not coincide perfectly. In addition, large tumors need overlapping ablations to achieve a necrosis large enough to cover the entire tumor and to avoid remnants of viable tumor tissue in a treated lesion [27].

While a large area of necrosis is desirable to completely include the treated lesion, thermal damaging of the calices and renal pelvis has to be

9 Renal Tumors

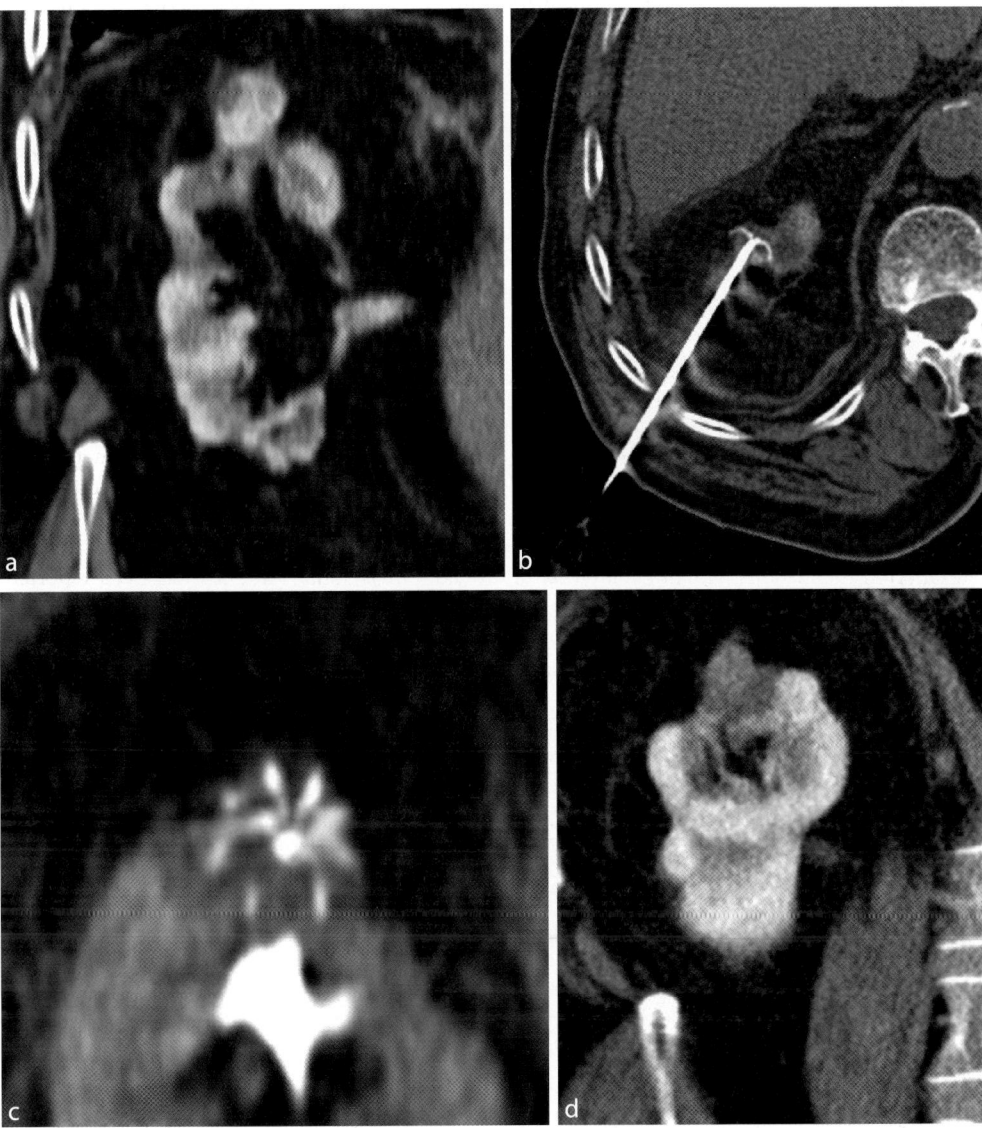

Fig. 9.1a–d A 74-year-old male patient with renal cell carcinoma and cardiovascular co-morbidity. Multiplanar reformat (MPR) from a preinterventional multislice spiral CT depicts an excentric 2.2-cm tumor at the upper pole of the right kidney (**a**). The patient was considered to be at high risk for surgery. The umbrella-shaped RF probe was introduced percutaneously via a dorsal approach (**b**). CT shows the tumor encompassed by the expanded prongs of the RF probe (**c**). One day after RFA, MPR from a contrast-enhanced MSCT shows a hypodense tumor without contrast enhancement, corresponding to complete tumor necrosis (**d**). A sufficient safety margin without contrast enhancement is visible

avoided in any case. Therefore, the ideal tumor for RF ablation is located peripherally with exophytic growth (Fig. 9.2), while centrally located tumors are considered a relative contraindication for thermal tumor ablation. However, in selected cases even centrally located RCCs may be treated successfully with RFA (Fig. 9.1). Moreover, in central tumors incomplete coagulation necrosis

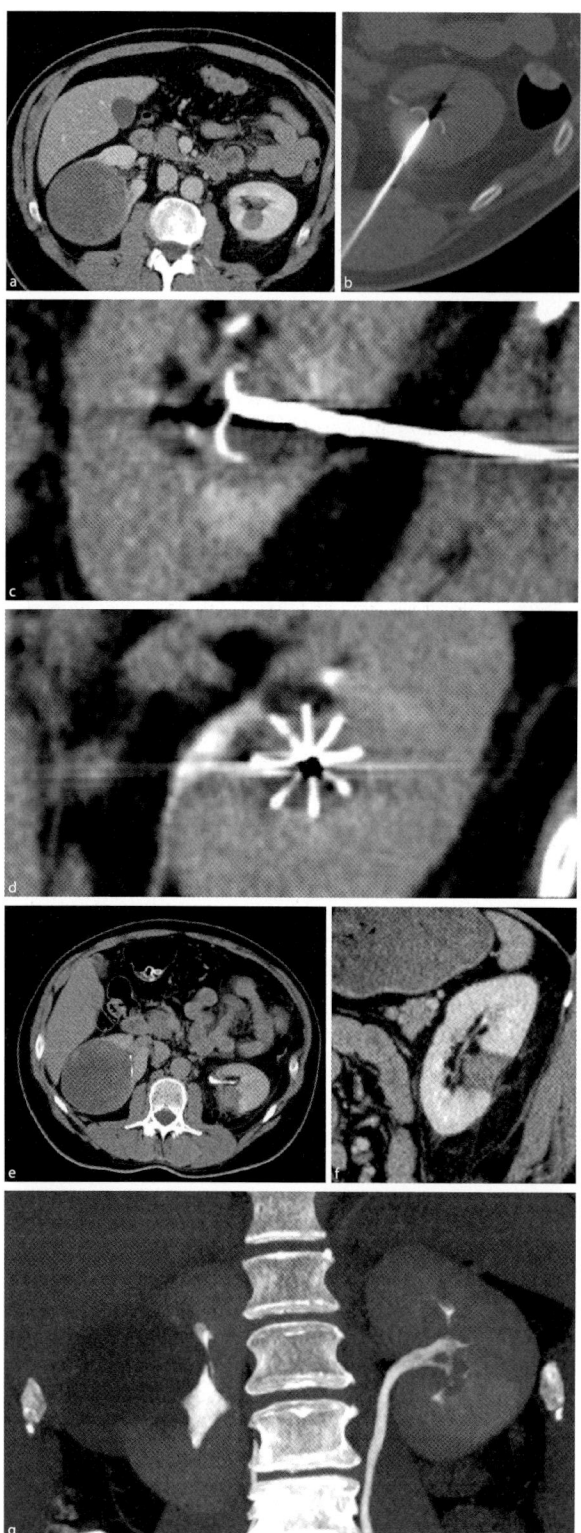

Fig. 9.2a–g A 50-year old male patient with double-sided papillary renal cell carcinoma. CT depicts a large tumor in the right kidney that was treated later by nephrectomy and a smaller central tumor on the left side (**a**). The tumor on the left was treated by RFA with the probe inserted via a mediodorsal approach (**b**). Multiplanar reformats from CT images obtained during the procedure show RF probe centrally positioned in the tumor (**c, d**). Postinterventional spiral CT including MPRs shows the wedge-shaped necrosis (**e, f**). CT urography excludes injury of the renal pelvis (**g**)

is more likely to occur because of a heat sink effect caused by large vessels [28]. To avoid damage to neighboring structures such as the colon, pararenal injection of air, CO2, water, or saline might be useful [29]. If needed, infusion of cold saline into the collecting system of the kidney may also be considered to avoid thermal damage of the renal pelvis [30]. The presence of a tumor thrombus is considered a contraindication to renal RFA.

In combination with tumor location and different probe designs, the heat sink effect has to be considered while planning the ablation procedure. As known from animal experiments, modulation of the local blood flow improves the efficiency of a RFA [17, 19]. Tumor embolization with coils or particles prior to RFA reduces the blood flow in the parenchyma adjacent to the embolized tissue and therefore results in better and more homogeneous heat distribution. Furthermore, embolization adds a therapeutic effect on its own. As a consequence, devascularizaion of hypervascularized renal tumors exceeding a diameter of 3 cm by embolization seems to be advantageous, as less energy is required and the remaining parenchyma will be protected [31–33]. To achieve optimal efficacy of a combined procedure, both interventions should be performed within 24 hs.

Unlike open or laparoscopic surgery, thermal therapy allows no direct visual control of the critical structures during the intervention. Consequently, an optimal monitoring system (US, CT, or MRI) is mandatory. While placement of the probes is possible under US, CT, and MRI guidance, none of these modalities permits on-line monitoring of the ablation results. Only MR temperature mapping can allow for a real-time assessment of the heat distribution and thus for real-time monitoring of the intervention's success. However, the technology needed for online temperature mapping during RFA is not commercially available yet, although the basic principle for temperature mapping in radiofrequency ablation has been described previously. The use of US during and immediately following the intervention is limited by the formation of microbubbles [34]. As coagulated and necrotic tissue is not perfused, administration of contrast material before probe retraction helps estimate the ablation result during CT- or MRI-guided RFA. For MRI, this technique allows for differentiation between treated and untreated renal parenchyma within a range of 2 mm [35].

RFA of renal masses can be performed with i.v. analgosedation as an outpatient procedure or, at most, requires overnight inpatient observation. In some centers, RFA is performed under general anesthesia, which ensures optimal patient compliance and comfort. It is common practice to perform biopsy prior to ablation, as biopsy results may affect subsequent patient management. The need and frequency of imaging follow-up may differ based on whether a mass is a histologically proven RCC or a benign tumor such as oncocytoma or angiomyolipoma [36]. In the literature, the timing suggested for biopsy varies. We recommend performing biopsy directly prior to RFA in order to perform tract ablation after the procedure and thereby avoid tumor seeding along the puncture tract, which is a known risk in biopsy of RCC.

After the intervention, it is important to follow stringent imaging surveillance to detect local or systemic recurrence. In general, contrast-enhanced CT or MRI are recommended for follow-up. Typical imaging findings in successfully treated renal tumors include a lack of contrast enhancement, shrinkage, and occasional retraction from normal parenchyma by fat infiltration [37]. While the optimal timing of imaging following RFA remains to be determined, it is agreed that an early evaluation is needed to assess for residual tumor, as this can be treated successfully by repeated percutaneous RFA. If no viable tumor is demonstrated, subsequent scans are generally performed at 3 months, 6 months, and every year.

9.4 Results and Complications

The first case of percutaneous RFA prior to radical open nephrectomy of an exophytic RCC was reported by Zlotta et al. in 1997 [12]. Histopathologic evaluation of the operation specimen revealed stromal edema and pyknosis. The zones of ablation were correctly predicted from the needle deployment. No viable tumor cells were demonstrated in the percutaneously treated tumor. In 1999, the first case of RFA as sole treatment for a renal tumor with 3 months of follow-up was reported [38]. Since then, the increasing number of reports on renal RFA outlines the potential of RFA for minimally invasive treatment of RCC. In addition, percutaneous radiofrequency ablation proved to be less costly than open or laparoscopic partial nephrectomy [39].

A large series with 34 patients with 42 RCCs undergoing 54 percutaneous RFA treatments was reported by Gervais et al. in 2003 [28]. The tumor size ranged from 1.1 to 8.9 cm, with a mean diameter of 3.2 cm. With a mean follow-up period of 13.2 months, this study proved RFA to be effective. Most important, this study firstly identified relevant factors for success of the ablation procedure. While parenchymal and central tumors recur more frequently if the diameter exceeds 3 cm, exophytic tumors can be treated effectively, even if they are bigger than 3 cm in diameter. Clinical results of renal RFA are summarized in Table 9.1.

Complications are rare and include hematoma, urinoma, infarction, ureteral obstruction, and cutaneous fistulas [40]. Most of these complications can be treated conservatively. Gervais et al. reported a complication rate of 7% with minor complications such as bladder outlet obstruction due to hematuria in prostatic hyperplasia, ureteral obstruction that required ureteral stent placement and perirenal hematoma [28]. Unlike hepatic or pulmonary RFA, in renal RF ablation a single 5-mm cutaneous metastasis along the puncture tract was reported; it was resected with no complications [41]. This type of complication, however, can be avoided by coagulation of the puncture tract during RF probe withdrawal. When compared to other thermal ablation techniques, the ability to avoid tract bleeding and tumor seeding by coagulating the puncture channel is an important advantage of RFA. Consequently, the risk of bleeding complications is low. Furthermore, animal experiments indicate an influence of tumor location on complication rate, with central tumors being prone to major complications, including renal artery injury [42].

Some investigators raised concern regarding the efficiency of renal RF ablation with respect to complete tumor necrosis. On histology, Michaels et al. found viable tumor in all but one specimen of the tumors included in this study [43]. Rendon et al. found viable residual tumor in four of five tumors undergoing partial or radical nephrectomy immediately after RFA and in three of five tumors undergoing nephrectomy 1 week after RFA [44]. Walther et al. reported one tumor with residual viable cells in 11 RCCs treated with RFA prior to surgical resection, whereas the remaining ten tumors were completely necrotic [45]. These observations have to be taken seriously, but there are methodological problems with some of the studies. Michaels's study group omitted overlapping ablations and did not correlate the results with imaging findings. Rendon et al. based their conclusions on viability solely on hematoxylin and eosin staining instead of the required reference standard of NADHase stains. As a consequence, these studies are contradicted by the results of other investigators. Jacomides et al. performed tumor resection secondary to RFA in 5 of 17 laparoscopically treated RCCs and did not find residual tumor on histology [46]. These observations, however, underscore the importance of scrupulous technique in performing RFA in patients suffering from RCC.

9.5 Alternative Thermal Ablation Techniques

Cryoablation is the oldest among all the minimally invasive ablation methods. This technique was first described for percutaneous ablation of renal tissue in 1995 [47]. The mechanism of tissue destruction is complex and contains immediate and delayed effects [48, 49]. Using liquid argon or liquid nitrogen temperatures of $-187\,°C$ or $-195\,°C$ are achieved at the tip of the cryoprobe. This results in the creation of an ice ball at the tip of the probe with the ice ball's volume depending on the diameter of the cryoprobe. As a consequence, tumors exceeding 2 cm in size require large (>3 mm) or multiple cryoprobes. With increasing size and number of the cryoprobes used in an intervention, the risk for bleeding increases. As the cold does not coagulate blood vessels, hemostyptic techniques have to be applied. Therefore, at present percutaneous cryotherapy is limited to small tumors. Lesions with a diameter above 2 cm need a surgical approach with the majority of all renal cryoablations being performed via a laparoscopic or an open surgery

Table 9.1 Survey on clinical RFA in renal cell carcinoma

Author/year	Method	Patients/tumors	Mean size (cm)	Local tumor control	Follow-up (months)
Zlotta et al. 1997 [12]	Perc. US, OP	2/3	2–5	3/3	N.A.
Walther et al. 2000 [45]	Open	4/11	2.2	10/11	N.A.
Michaels et al. 2002 [43]	Open US, OP	15/20	2,4	1/20	N.A.
Ogan et al. 2002 [63]	Perc. CT	12/13	2.4	12/13	4.9
Matlaga et al. 2002 [64]	Open US, OP	10/10	3.2	8/10	N.A.
Pavlovich et al. 2002 [65]	Perc. US, CT	21/24	2.4	24/24	2
de Baere et al. 2002 [66]	Perc. US/CT	5/5	3–4	5/5	9
Rendon et al. 2002 [44]	Lap./perc., OP	10/11	2.4	4/11	N.A.
Roy-Choudhury et al. 2002 [67]	Perc. US/CT	12/15	3.0	11/15	13.6
Jacomides et al. 2003 [46]	Lap. all, 5 OP	13/17	2	17/17	9.8
Su et al. 2003 [68]	Perc. CT	29/35	2.2	35/35	9
Mayo-Smith et al. 2003 [41]	Perc. US/CT	32/32	2.6	31/32	9
Farrell et al. 2003 [69]	Perc., OP US/CT	20/35	1.7	35/35	9
Lewin et al. 2004 [70]	Perc. MRI	10/10	2.6	10/10	23
Zagoria et al. 2004 [71]	Perc. CT	22/24	3.5	20/22	7
Veltri et al. 2004 [72]	Perc. US	13/18	2.5	16/18	14
Mahnken et al. 2005 [33]	Perc CT	14/15	3.0	15/15	13.9
Chiou YY et al. 2005 [73]	Perc.	12/12	3.7	9/12	–
Matsumoto et al. 2005[a] [74]	Perc. CT, lap.	91/109	2.4	109/109	–
Gervais et al. 2005 [20]	Perc. CT/US	85/100	3.2	89/100	28
Total/mean		432/519	2.7	89.8%	11.7

Perc., percutaneous; lap., laparoscopic; OP, surgical; US, ultrasound; CT, computed tomography; MRI, magnetic resonance imaging; N.A., not applicable
[a] Includes 15 benign tumors

approach [50, 51]. However, percutaneous renal cryotherapy has successfully been performed by several investigators. Shingleton et al. used an interventional MRI system for percutaneous MRI-guided probe placement and monitoring of the intervention [52]. Percutaneous cryotherapy is also feasible with real-time monitoring using an open MR scanner [53]. The main advantage of this technique is the direct visualization of the ice ball and therefore online assessment of treatment success.

LITT has also been shown to be a viable treatment option in RCC. This technique involves the placement of laser fibers in the tumor, followed by thermal ablation of the target tissue by applying laser energy. Diode (830–980 nm) and Nd:YAG (1040 nm) lasers have been used for thermal ablation of renal parenchyma [54]. However, for lesions exceeding 2 cm in diameter, a cooling catheter is necessary, which increases the diameter of the device up to 9F. LITT is principally MRI-compatible and permits MRI thermometry during ablation. Thus, this technique is well suited for MRI-guided interventions. However, the technical expertise required of LITT is greater than that of RFA or cryotherapy. Consequently, there is only a small number of clinical reports available, which are limited to patients with unresectable tumors [55, 56].

Microwave ablation is characterized by rapid induction of small necrosis volumes. So far this ablation technique has been used intraoperatively only. Although technically very interesting, there are no microwave probes available that are suited for percutaneous induction of thermal lesions with a diameter of more than 2 cm. A major advantage of this technique is its ability to avoid bleeding from the renal parenchyma incision. Nevertheless, there are only little clinical data published on this treatment option [57, 58].

High-intensity focused ultrasound is the least invasive of all the available thermal ablative therapies. This technique has successfully been used to create renal coagulation necrosis [59]. Only recently, preliminary experience in has been reported from patient studies [60–62]. Still, this technique is considered experimental, with several problems concerning visualization of the target lesion as well as control of the lesion size.

9.6 Summary

The treatment of RCC is rapidly changing. The introduction of minimally invasive thermal ablation techniques offers a safe and accurate alternative to open surgery in the treatment of renal tumors. Because of its technical benefits, percutaneous radiofrequency ablation took the lead among these minimally invasive techniques. Supported by convincing results from experimental studies, patient data prove this procedure to be safe and efficient. As a minimally invasive and nephron-sparing technique, it is well suited for patients with a single kidney, multiple tumors, or contraindications for open surgery.

References

1. Jemal A, Tiwari R, Murray T, Ghafoor A, Samuels A, Ward E, Feuer EJ, Thun M (2004) Cancer statistics, 2004. CA Cancer J Clin 54:8–29
2. Pantuck AJ, Zisman A, Belldegrun AS (2001) The changing natural history of renal cell carcinoma. J Urol 166:297–301
3. Homma Y, Kawabe K, Kitamura T, Nishimura Y, Shinohara M, Kondo Y, Saito I, Minowada S, Asakage Y (1995) Increased incidental detection and reduced mortality in renal cancer – recent retrospective analysis at eight institutions. Int J Urol 2:77–80
4. Zagoria RJ, Dyer RB (1998) The small renal mass: detection, characterization, and management. Abdom Imaging 23:256–265
5. Guinan PD, Vogelzang NJ, Fremgen AM, Chmiel JS, Sylvester JL, Sener SF, Imperato JP (1995) Renal cell carcinoma: tumor size, stage and survival. Members of the Cancer Incidence and End Results Committee. J Urol 153:901–903
6. Thrasher JB, Paulson DF (1993) Prognostic factors in renal cancer. Urol Clin North Am 20:247–262
7. Vogelzang NJ, Stadler WM (1988) Kidney cancer. Lancet 352:1691–1696
8. Uzzo RG, Novick AC (2001) Nephron sparing surgery for renal tumors: indications techniques and outcomes. J Urol 166:6–18
9. Fergany AF, Hafez KS, Novick AC (2000) Long-term results of nephron-sparing surgery for localized renal cell carcinoma: 10-year follow up. J Urol 163:442–445
10. Herr HW (1999) Partial nephrectomy for unilateral renal cell carcinoma and a normal contralateral kidney: 10-year follow-up. J Urol 1161:33–35
11. Moll V, Becht E, Ziegler M (1993) Kidney preserving surgery in renal cell tumors: indications, techniques and results in 152 patients. J Urol 150:319–323
12. Zlotta AR, Wildschutz T, Raviv G, Peny MO, van Gansbeke D, Noel JC, Schulman CC (1997) Radiofrequency interstitial tumor ablation (RITA) is a possible new modality for treatment of renal cancer: ex vivo and in vivo experience. J Endourol 11:251–258
13. Munver R, Threatt CB, Delvecchio FC, Preminger GM, Polascik TJ (2002) Hypertonic saline-augmented radiofrequency ablation of the VX-2 tumor implanted in the rabbit kidney: a short-term survival pilot study. Urology 60:170–175
14. Hsu TH, Fidler ME, Gill IS (2000) Radiofrequency ablation of the kidney: acute and chronic histology in porcine model. Urol 56:872–875
15. Crowley JD, Shelton J, Iverson AJ, Burton MP, Dalrymple NC, Bishoff JT (2000) Laparoscopic and computed tomography-guided percutaneous radiofrequency ablation of renal tissue: acute and chronic effects in an animal model. Urology 57:976–980
16. Polascik TJ, Hamper U, Lee BR, Dai Y, Hilton J, Magee CA, Crone JK, Shue MJ, Ferrell M, Trapanotto V, Adiletta M, Partin AW (1999) Ablation of renal tumors in a rabbit model with interstitial saline-augmented radiofrequency energy: preliminary report of a new technology. Urology 53:465–472

17. Aschoff AJ, Sulman A, Martinez M, Duerk JL, Resnick MI, MacLennan GT, Lewin JS (2001) Perfusion-modulated MR imaging-guided radiofrequency ablation of the kidney in a porcine model. AJR Am J Roentgenol 177:151–158
18. Chang I, Mikityansky I, Wray-Cahen D, Pritchard WF, Karanian JW, Wood BJ (2004) Effects of perfusion on radiofrequency ablation in swine kidneys. Radiology 231:500–505
19. Corwin TS, Lindberg G, Traxer O, Gettman MT, Smith TG, Pearle MS, Cadeddu JA (2001) Laparoscopic radiofrequency thermal ablation of renal tissue with and without hilar occlusion. J Urol 166:281–284
20. Gervais DA, McGovern FJ, Arellano RS, McDougal WS, Mueller PR (2005) Radiofrequency ablation of renal cell carcinoma: part 1, indications, results, and role in patient management over a 6-year period and ablation of 100 tumors. AJR Am J Roentgenol 185:64–71
21. Neeman Z, Sarin S, Coleman J, Fojo T, Wood BJ (2005) Radiofrequency ablation for tumor-related massive hematuria. J Vasc Interv Radiol 16:417–421
22. Brown SD, Vansonnenberg E, Morrison PR, Diller L, Shamberger RC (2005) CT-guided radiofrequency ablation of pediatric Wilms tumor in a solitary kidney. Pediatr Radiol 39:923–928
23. Zagoria RJ, Chen MY, Kavanagh PV, Torti FM (2001) Radio frequency ablation of lung metastases from renal cell carcinoma. J Urol 166:1827–1828
24. Gervais DA, Arellano RS, Mueller PR (2002) Percutaneous radiofrequency ablation of nodal metastases. Cardiovasc Intervent Radiol 25:547–549
25. Goetz MP, Callstrom MR, Charboneau JW, Farrell MA, Maus TP, Welch TJ, Wong GY, Sloan JA, Novotny PJ, Petersen IA, Beres RA, Regge D, Capanna R, Saker MB, Gronemeyer DH, Gevargez A, Ahrar K, Choti MA, de Baere TJ, Rubin J (2004) Percutaneous image-guided radiofrequency ablation of painful metastases involving bone: a multicenter study. J Clin Oncol 22:300–306
26. Goldberg SN, Gazelle GS, Mueller PR (2000) Thermal ablation therapy for focal malignancy: a unified approach to underlying principles, techniques, and diagnostic imaging guidance. AJR Am J Ronetgenol 174:323–331
27. Rendon RA, Kachura JR, Sweet JM, Gertner MR, Sherar MD, Robinette M, Tsihlias J, Trachtenberg J, Sampson H, Jewett MA (2002) The uncertainty of radio frequency treatment of renal cell carcinoma: findings at immediate and delayed nephrectomy. J Urol 167:1587–1592
28. Gervais DA, McGovern FJ, Arellano RS, McDougal SW, Mueller PR (2003) Renal cell carcinoma: clinical experience and technical success with radio-frequency ablation of 42 tumors. Radiology 226:417–424
29. Farrell MA, Charboneau JW, Callstrom MR, Reading CC, Engen DE, Blute ML (2003) Paranephric water instillation: a technique to prevent bowel injury during percutaneous renal radiofrequency ablation. AJR Am J Roentgenol 181:1315–1317
30. Schultze D, Morris CS, Bhave AD, Worgan BA, Najarian KE (2003) Radiofrequency ablation of renal transitional cell carcinoma with protective cold saline infusion. J Vasc Interv Radiol 14:489–492
31. Hall WH, McGahan JP, Link DP, deVere White RW (2000) Combined embolization and percutaneous radiofrequency ablation of a solid renal tumor. AJR Am J Roentgenol 174:1592–1594
32. Tacke J, Mahnken A, Bucker A, Rohde D, Gunther RW (2001) Nephron-sparing percutaneous ablation of a 5 cm renal cell carcinoma by superselective embolization and percutaneous RF ablation. Rofo 173:980–983
33. Mahnken A, Rohde D, Brkovic D, Günther RW, Tacke J (2005) Percutaneous radiofrequency ablation of renal cell carcinoma: preliminary results. Acta Radiol 46:208–214
34. Rendon RA, Gertner MR, Sherar MD, Asch MR, Kachura JR, Sweet J, Jewett MA (2001) Development of a radiofrequency based thermal therapy technique in an in vivo porcine model for the treatment of small renal masses. J Urol 166:292–298
35. Merkle EM, Shonk JR, Duerk JL, Jacobs GH, Lewin JS (1999) MR-guided RF thermal ablation of the kidney in a porcine model. AJR Am J Roentgenol 173:645–651
36. Tuncali K, vanSonnenberg E, Shankar S, Mortele KJ, Cibas ES, Silverman SG (2004) Evaluation of patients referred for percutaneous ablation of renal tumors: importance of a preprocedural diagnosis. AJR Am J Roentgenol 183:575–582
37. Matsumoto ED, Watumull L, Johnson DB, Ogan K, Taylor GD, Josephs S, Cadeddu JA (2004) The radiographic evolution of radio frequency ablated renal tumors. J Urol 172:45–48

38. McGovern FJ, Goldberg SN, Wood BJ, Mueller PR (1999) Radiofrequency ablation of renal cell carcinoma via image-guided needle electrodes. J Urol 161:599–600
39. Lotan Y Cadeddu JA (2005) A cost comparison of nephron-sparing surgical techniques for renal tumour. BJU Int 95:1039–1042
40. Rhim H, Dodd GD, Chintapalli KN, Wood BJ, Dupuy DE, Hvizda JL, Sewell PE, Goldberg SN (2004) Radiofrequency thermal ablation of abdominal tumors: lessons learned from complications. Radiographics 24:41–52
41. Mayo-Smith WW, Dupuy DE, Parikh PM, Pezzullo JA, Cronan JJ (2003) Imaging-guided percutaneous radiofrequency ablation of solid renal masses: techniques and outcomes of 38 treatment sessions in 32 consecutive patients. AJR Am J Roentgenol 180:1503–1508
42. Lee JM, Kim SW, Chung GH, Lee SY, Han YM, Kim CS (2003) Open radio-frequency thermal ablation of renal VX2 tumors in a rabbit model using a cooled-tip electrode: feasibility, safety, and effectiveness. Eur Radiol 13:1324–1332
43. Michaels MJ, Rhee HK, Mourtzinos AP, Summerhayes IC, Silverman ML, Libertino JA (2002) Incomplete renal tumor destruction using radio frequency interstitial ablation. J Urol 168:2406–2410
44. Rendon RA, Kachura JR, Sweet JM, Gertner MR, Sherar MD, Robinette M, Trachtenberg JTJ, Sampson H, Jewett MAS (2002) The uncertainty of radiofrequency treatment of renal cell carcinoma: findings at immediate and delayed nephrectomy. J Urol 167:1587–1592
45. Walther MM, Shawker TH, Libutti SK, Lubensky I, Choyke PL, Venzon D, Linehan WM (2000) A phase 2 study of radio frequency interstitial tissue ablation of localized renal tumors. J Urol 163:1424–1427
46. Jacomides L, Ogan K, Watumull L, Cadeddu JA (2003) Laparoscopic application of radio frequency energy enables in situ renal tumor ablation and partial nephrectomy. J Urol 169:49–53
47. Uchida M, Imaide Y, Sugimoto K, Uehara H, Watanabe H (1995) Percutaneous cryosurgery for renal tumors. Br J Urol 75:132–136
48. Hoffmann NE, Bischof JC (2002) The cryobiology of cryosurgical injury. Urology 60 [2 Suppl 1]:40–49
49. Stephenson RA, King DK, Rohr LR (1996) Renal cryoablation in a canine model. Urology 47:772–776
50. Nadler RB, Kim SC, Rubenstein JN, Yap RL, Campbell SC, User HM (2003) Laparoscopic renal cryosurgery: the northwestern experience. J Urol 170:1121–1125
51. Korshandi M, Foy RC, Chong W, Hoenig D, Cohen JK, Rukstalis DB (2002) Preliminary experience with cryoablation of renal lesions smaller than 4 centimeters. J Am Osteopath Assoc 102:277–281
52. Shingleton WB, Sewell PE (2001) Percutaneous renal tumor cryoablation with MRI guidance. J Urol 165:773–776
53. Harada J, Dohi M, Mogami T (2001) Initial experience of percutaneous renal cryosurgery under the guidance of horizontal open MRI system. Radiat Med 19:291–296
54. Lofti MA, McCue P, Gomella LG (1994) Laparoscopic interstitial contact laser ablation of renal lesions: an experimental model. J Endourol 8:153–156
55. Dick EA, Joarder R, De Jode MG, Wragg P, Vale JA, Gedroyc WM (2002) Magnetic resonance imaging-guided laser thermal ablation of renal tumours. BJU Int 90:814–822
56. De Jode MG, Vale JA, Gedroyc WM (1999) MR-guided laser thermoablation of inoperable renal tumors in an open-configuration interventional MR scanner: preliminary clinical experience in three cases. J Magn Reson Imaging 10:545–549
57. Hirao Y, Fujimoto K, Yoshii M, Tanaka N, Hayashi Y, Momose H, Samma S, Okajima E, Uemura H, Yoshida K, Ozono S (2002) Non-ischemic nephron-sparing surgery for small renal cell carcinoma: complete tumor enucleation using a microwave tissue coagulator. Jpn J Clin Oncol 32:95–102
58. Murota T, Kawakita M, Oguchi N, Shimada O, Danno S, Fujita I, Matsuda T (2002) Retroperitoneoscopic partial nephrectomy using microwave coagulation for small renal tumors. Eur Urol 41:540–545
59. Paterson RF, Barret E, Siqueira TM Jr, Gardner TA, Tavakkoli J, Rao VV, Sanghvi NT, Cheng L, Shalhav AL (2003) Laparoscopic partial kidney ablation with high intensity focused ultrasound. J Urol 169:347–351

60. Susani M, Madersbacher S, Kratzik C, Vingers L, Marberger M (1993) Morphology of tissue destruction induced by focused ultrasound. Eur Urol 23:34–38
61. Kohrmann KU, Michel MS, Gaa J, Marlinghaus E, Alken P (2002) High intensity focused ultrasound as noninvasive therapy for multilocal renal cell carcinoma: case study and review of the literature. J Urol 167:2397–2403
62. Wu F, Wang ZB, Chen WZ, Bai J, Zhu H, Qiao TY (2003) Preliminary experience using high intensity focused ultrasound for the treatment of patients with advanced stage renal malignancy. J Urol 170:2237–2240
63. Ogan K, Jacomides L, Dolmatch BL, Rivera FJ, Dellaria MF, Josephs SC, Cadeddu JA (2002) Percutaneous radiofrequency ablation of renal tumors: technique, limitations, and morbidity. Urology 60:954–958
64. Matlaga BR, Zagoria RJ, Woodruff RD, Torti FM, Hall MC (2002) Phase II trial of radio frequency ablation of renal cancer: evaluation of the kill zone. J Urol 168:2401–2405
65. Pavlovich CP, Walther MM, Choyke PL, Pautler SE, Chang R, Linehan WM, Wood BJ (2002) Percutaneous radio frequency ablation of small renal tumors: initial results. J Urol 167:10–15
66. De Baere T, Kuoch V, Smayra T, Dromain C, Cabrera T, Court B, Roche A (2002) Radiofrequency ablation of renal cell carcinoma: preliminary clinical experience. Urology 167:1961–1964
67. Roy-Choudhury SH, Cast JE, Lee-Elliott CE, Breen DJ (2002) Percutaneous radiofrequency (RFA) ablation of small renal cell carcinoma (RCC) – medium-term outcome (abstract). Radiology 225:S387
68. Su LM, Jarrett TW, Chan DY, Kavoussi LR, Solomon SB (2003) Percutaneous computed tomography-guided radiofrequency ablation of renal masses in high surgical risk patients: preliminary results. Urology 61 [Suppl 4A]:26–33
69. Farrell MA, Charboneau WJ, DiMarco DS, Chow GK, Zincke H, Callstrom MR, Lewis BD, Lee RA, Reading CC (2003) Imaging-guided radiofrequency ablation of solid renal tumors. AJR Am J Roentgenol 180:1509–1513
70. Lewin JS, Nour SG, Connell CF, Sulman A, Duerk JL, Resnick MI, Haaga JR (2004) Phase II clinical trial of interactive MR imaging-guided interstitial radiofrequency thermal ablation of primary kidney tumors: initial experience. Radiology 232:835–845
71. Zagoria RJ, Hawkins AD, Clark PE, Hall MC, Matlaga BR, Dyer RB, Chen MY (2004) Percutaneous CT-guided radiofrequency ablation of renal neoplasms: factors influencing success. AJR Am J Roentgenol 183:201–207
72. Veltri A, De Fazio G, Malfitana V, Isolato G, Fontana D, Tizzani A, Gandini G (2004) Percutaneous US-guided RF thermal ablation for malignant renal tumors: preliminary results in 13 patients. Eur Radiol 14:2303–2310
73. Chiou YY, Hwang JI, Chou YH, Wang JH, Chiang JH, Chang CY (2005) Percutaneous radiofrequency ablation of renal cell carcinoma. J Chin Med Assoc 68:221–225
74. Matsumoto ED, Johnson DB, Ogan K, Trimmer C, Sagalowsky A, Margulis V, Cadeddu JA (2005) Short-term efficacy of temperature-based radiofrequency ablation of small renal tumors. Urology 65:877–881

10 Thermal Ablation in Bone Tumors

Bernhard Gebauer, Per-Ulf Tunn

10.1 Introduction

In the past decade, percutaneous image-guided therapy of various soft tissue tumors has received significant attention. In particular microtherapy of hepatic lesions by thermoablation has extended throughout the world and is actually the best investigated field of percutaneous image-guided microtherapy. Most thermal ablative techniques use heat to destroy the cellular structures causing scarring. Heating energy could be generated by laser energy, radiofrequency, microwave, or high-focused ultrasound.

The nature of thermal damage by heating depends on the tissue temperature reached and the duration. Cells become more sensitive to systemic chemotherapy or radiation when their temperature in increased to 42 °C (e.g., hyperthermia); heating cells to 45 °C for several hours produces irreversible cellular damage. Further heating the cells to 50–55 °C shortens the necessary time to irreversible cell damage to 4–6 min. Nearly immediate coagulation of tissue and cells could be achieved with temperatures between 60 and 100 °C. At more than 100–110 °C, vaporization and carbonization of tissue leads to impedance increment [1]. The diameter of coagulation necrosis achieved from thermal ablation is equivalent to the energy deposited into the tissue multiplied by local tissue interactions (organ and tumor blood flow, electric and thermal conductivity) minus heat loss (conductive and convective): this approximation is called the bioheat transfer equation [2, 3].

Laser-induced interstitial thermotherapy (LITT) and radiofrequency ablation (RFA) are the most frequently used techniques in thermal ablation. In LITT, tissue necrosis is induced by the heating effect of a coherent, monochromatic light. The most commonly used laser is a neodymium yttrium aluminum garnet (Nd:YAG) laser system with 1,064-nm wavelength. The infrared low-power (3–15 W) laser light is delivered through a thin (400 µm in diameter) quartz fiberoptic with a disperse tip [4]. Simple laser fibers produce a 1 cm destruction in diameter, so cooled applicators have been developed, which prevent carbonization at the laser optic tip and allow greater tissue penetration and tissue ablations up to 5 cm in diameter [5, 6].

Radiofrequency ablation (RFA) is an electrosurgical technique [7]. Alternating current between the ground pads and an intratumoral applicator causes movement of irons in the tissue, which results in frictional heating of the tissue surrounding the applicator tip [8, 9]. As in laser thermoablation, carbonization of tissue surrounding the applicator tip reduces ablation size to 1 cm in diameter in simple systems. To overcome this limitation, slow or pulsed heating generators and multipolar applicator systems have been developed. Another approach is to modify the applicator design, e.g., multiprobe array electrodes, internally cooled electrodes, or continuous saline infusion [10–13]. With these improvements, ablations up to 5–7 cm in diameter can be achieved.

Microwave hyperthermia is an alternative thermoablative method [14, 15]. The high frequency of the electromagnetic radiation (30 MHz to 30 GHz) around the applicator leads to heating the intracellular water and consecutive coagulation necrosis. In contrast to RFA and LITT, the tissue penetration of the heat is reduced, and no larger series of microwave ablation in skeletal lesions have been published.

High-intensity focused ultrasound (HIFU) is the only true percutaneous technique for thermal ablation, because no applicator need be introduced into the tissue [16, 17]. The intensity of ultrasound waves in HIFU is up to 1000 times greater than in diagnostic ultrasound and the waves cause vibration and frictional forces in the tissue, resulting in tissue heating and coagulative necrosis. Although HIFU treatments of osteosarcoma and soft tissue sarcoma are published, in general skeletal lesions are not suitable for ultrasound ablation, because, as in diagnostic ultrasound, the cortical bone absorbs or reflects the ultrasound beams [18].

Skeletal lesions suitable for microinvasive therapy are mainly definitive treatment of osteoid osteomas, benign lesions with typical pain that worsens at night, and palliative therapy of symptomatic bone metastasis without palliation to standard therapy.

10.2 Osteoid Osteoma

Osteoid osteoma (Oo) is a painful benign osteoblastic bone tumor, composed of osteoblasts and an osteoid forming a small (usually < 15 mm) radiolucent nidus. This tumor was first described by Jaffe in 1935 [19]. The nidus is surrounded by an osteoblastic wall with increased neural and arterial supply. Additionally Oos produce prostaglandins with local inflammatory effects and vasodilatation. Both are assumed to be responsible for the typical pain of osteoid osteomas, which worsens at night and shows a quick relief after blockade of the arachidonic pathway by antiphlogistics [20]. Increased blood supply boosts bone growth in the area around the nidus and often causes synovitis.

Oos are responsible for approximately 10% of all primary bone tumors and mainly develop in children and young adults, with a male predominance. The corticalis of long bones (tibia, femur, humerus, radius, or ulna) and the vertebral spine are the typical tumor locations. Because Oos have a typical pain that resolves after oral non-steroidal anti-inflammatory drugs (NSAIDs), a typical location and patient age, and a typical X-ray appearance, most authors resign to a preinterventional histology in a typical constellation. Furthermore, biopsies in Oos are often nondiagnostic, even after surgery [21, 22].

Oos may undergo spontaneous regression after several years of conservative management, but they may cause other symptoms, such as growth disturbance, bone deformity, and painful scoliosis [23]. Chronic use of NSAIDs could cause additional side effects, especially gastrointestinal. Conventional treatment of Oos consists of en-bloc resection of the nidus. Unfortunately, the nidal area is often difficult to localize in the operating room, even with fluoroscopy, so a large resection, which is disproportional to the lesion size, is necessary [24]. In addition, wider surgical resection often requires internal fixation and/or bone grafting. Postoperative pain persists in 7%–20% of cases, Oo recurs in 7%–12%, and complications such as fractures, infections, and pain from the implants occur in 9%–28% of cases [25–27].

Several minimally invasive techniques with computed tomography (CT) guidance (guided resection, guided nidal drilling, guided ethanol injection, and guided thermal ablation) for Oo have been developed. Image-guided thermal ablation has emerged as the most common form of percutaneous Oo treatment.

Rosenthal first described the thermal ablation of an Oo by radiofrequency in 1992 [28]. Table 10.1 gives an overview of the largest published series of thermal ablation in Oos, which shows a predominance of RFA induced thermal ablation. Spinal lesions near the medulla for thermal ablation are controversial. Some authors regard this location as a contraindication for thermal ablation, whereas others have published encouraging studies concerning this site [29–33]. In spinal osteoid osteomas, the indication for ablation should be carefully reviewed, dependent on the site and access route, other therapeutical alternatives, and on the personal skill of the interventional radiologist.

Usually the procedure of thermal ablation is performed with computed tomography (CT)

Table 10.1 Overview of MEDLINE published studies concerning thermoablation of osteoid osteoma sorted by number of patients

Author	N	Technique	Primary success	Residual or recurrent pain	Follow-up (months)
Rosenthal et al. 2003 [71]	117a	RFA	91% (107/117)	5% (6/117)	NS
Rimondi et al. 2005 [72]	97	RFA	84.5% (82/97)	15.5% (15/97)	NS
Vanderschueren et al. 2002 [73]	97	RFA	76% (74/97)	24% (23/97)	41 (5–81)
Lindner et al. 2001 [74]	58	RFA	95% (55/58)	5% (3/58)	NS
Woertler et al. 2001 [75]	47	RFA	94% (44/47)	6% (3/47)	22
Cioni et al. 2004 [76]	38	RFA	79% (30/38)	21% (8/38)	12–66 (35.5)
Gangi et al. 1998 [77]	28	LITT	93% (26/28)	7% (2/28)	12
Witt et al. 2000 [78]	23	LITT	96% (22/23)	4% (1/23)	15
Ghanem et al. 2003 [79]	23	RFA	100% (23/23)	0% (0/23)	43
Gebauer et al. 2005 [80]	17 (RFA 8, LITT 12)	RFA/LITT	82.4% (14/17)	17.6% (3/17)	28 (4–51)
Gallazzi et al. 2001 [81]	15	RFA	93% (14/15)	7% (1/15)	NS
Barei et al. 2000 [82]	11	RFA	91% (10/11)	9% (1/11)	NS
Venbrux et al. 2003 [83]	9	RFA	56% (5/9)	44% (4/9)	10.3 (1–26)
Sequeiros et al. 2003 [84]	5	LITT	80% (4/5)	20% (1/5)	NS
Total (RFA/LITT)	588 (520/68)		86.7% (87%/91.1%)	12.1% (12.5%/9%)	

RFA, radiofrequency ablation; LITT, laser induced thermal therapy; NS, not stated
a Rosenthal et al. presented 271 ablation procedures in 263 patients. Only in 126 patients was follow-up data available; 117 of these had a prior, not otherwise (surgery, RFA) treated osteoid osteoma

guidance with the patient on general anesthesia. CT guidance is necessary to exactly localize the area of the nidus and to avoid damage to other surrounding tissues and structures. Most authors use a dedicated bone biopsy needle to drill into the nidus and use this channel for thermal applicator placement. Our experience favors power drilling of the nidus with a 2–3.5 mm drill, which is less time-consuming and exhausting, facilitates applicator placement, and is necessary if larger diameter applicators are used, as in water-cooled LITT ablation (Fig. 10.1).

Compared to other solid tumors (liver, lung, or kidney), Oos are relatively small and benign tumors, so no safety margin and only a small ablative zone around the applicator is necessary. An objective temperature of 90–100 °C with 3–5 min of ablation at an objective temperature is sufficient in RFA or LITT. The access route to the Oo passing sensitive tissues or structures could be protected by a drill sheath or by isolation with an angiography sheath.

The procedure can be done on an outpatient or short hospitalization basis. Usually the patient is discharged the same day following recovery from anesthesia. Normal daily activities can be resumed immediately, after ablation of lesions in weight-bearing bones, strenuous sports should be avoided for 8–12 weeks. Usually no cast, splint, crutches, or physical therapy is necessary.

After careful preoperative planning, technical success, which means the ability to enter and to ablate the nidus, is nearly certain. The primary success, complete relief of symptoms without the use of antiphlogistics 1 month after ablation, can usually be achieved in 80%–96% of cases

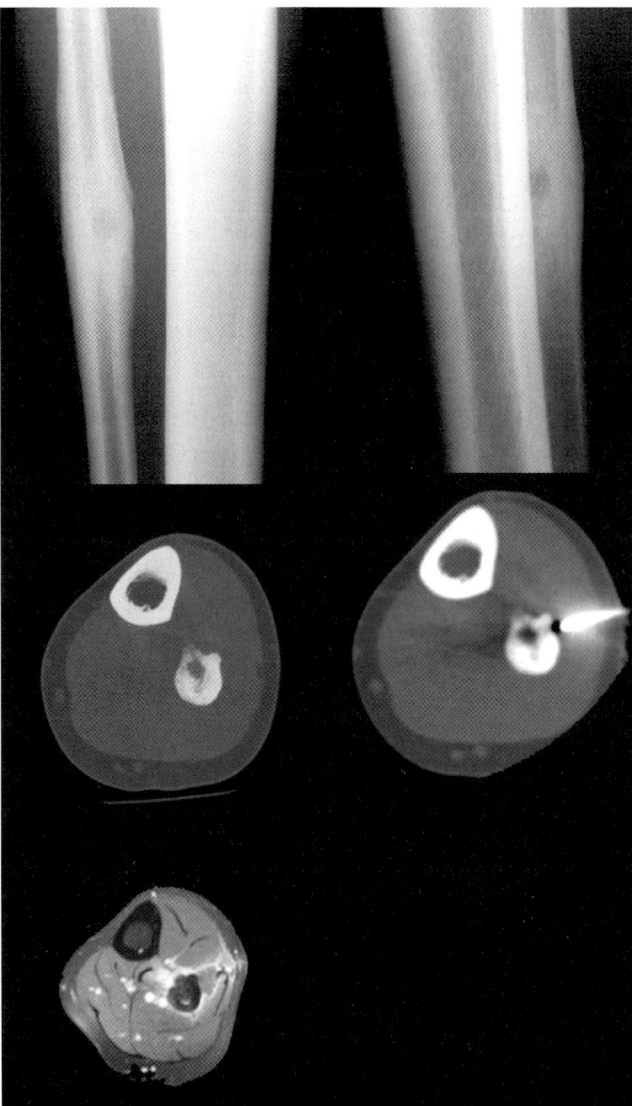

Fig. 10.1 Radiofrequency ablation of a fibular osteoid osteoma. Typical radiological osteoid osteoma with central radiolucent nidus, surrounded by a hyperostotic rim. Under CT guidance, power drilling from latero-ventral and radiofrequency ablation. Follow-up MRI (Fat-saturated T1-weighted image after contrast injection) 5 days after ablation without nidal enhancement, indicating a complete nidal ablation. Enhancement of preexistent periosteum, indicating hypervascularization and inflammation due to active osteoid osteoma. Small soft tissue burning near the bone, but no nerve impairment

(Table 10.1). Primary incomplete ablation with persistent pain after ablation was recorded in 4%–20%.

Recurrent pain, which has to be interpreted as an osteoid osteoma recurrence, occurs in 0%–20% of cases and can usually be successfully treated by a second ablation. Rosenthal et. al. compared surgical resection with radiofrequency ablation in 125 patients with osteoid osteoma [25]. Eighty-seven patients underwent surgical resection and 38 were treated by radiofrequency ablation. In an average time of 12 months (range, 5–17 months) after intervention, 9% of the surgical patients had recurrent pain and 12% of the radiofrequency patients. This difference was not statistically significant. The hospital stay for operative patients and those treated with RFA was 4.7 and 0.2 days, respectively. Of the surgery group, 30% had persistent symptoms, 23% in the RFA group. Two patients in the surgical group had major complications requiring five additional operations, whereas no major complications occurred in the RFA group.

Lindner et al. compared costs of treatment in different strategies in osteoid osteoma by adding procedural costs and costs stemming from the hospital stay and the treatment of complications. Social costs due to inactivity and disability were not considered in this study. Ninety-one patients were included in this study. Surgical costs were estimated at $13,826 for en-bloc resection, $10,857 for marginal nidus resection, and $10,992 for intralesional curettage. CT-guided therapies such as CT-guided nidus drilling was estimated at $8,589 and CT-guided RFA at $6,583. In this study, radiofrequency ablation was the most cost-effective treatment method and the method with the shortest rehabilitation period and in-patient treatment.

Another CT-guided method for treating osteoid osteoma is CT-guided nidus drilling and destruction. This technique needs no LITT or RFA equipment and no LITT or RFA applicator, a disposable item, but, because larger drills are necessary in CT-guided drilling, postinterventional morbidity is higher than with thermal ablation [34–36]. Other authors combined CT-guided drilling with ethanol injection into the nidus [37–39]. Ethanol, especially in high concentrations, has a cytotoxic effect on cell membranes and cells [40]. This effect is used in interventional therapy for percutaneous ethanol injection (PEI) in hepatocellular carcinoma, in plexus blockade therapy in uncontrollable epigastric pain or for sympatholysis. Ethanol destroys tissue cells and nerves and reduces transmission of pain. But the distribution of the injected ethanol cannot be precisely predicted. In the treatment of osteoid osteoma, the results of ethanol injection after nidal drilling were similar to simple CT-guided drilling.

Thermal ablation of osteoid osteoma by an experienced hand is a safe microtherapy, with complete ablation in 80%–94% of cases. In 4%–20%, a second ablation could be necessary. There is currently no consensus concerning thermal ablation of spinal lesions. Current data shows no difference between radiofrequency and laser-induced therapy in osteoid osteoma. Using whether RFA or LITT in osteoid osteoma should depend on personal and institutional experience and resources.

10.3 Symptomatic Bone Metastasis

In the US, nearly 1.3 million cases of cancer were diagnosed in 2001, 50% of which had the potential to spread to the musculoskeletal system [41, 42]. The preference of some malignancies to metastasize into the skeleton is still not understood. Liotta et al. suggested that 30% of the anatomic distribution of the metastasis can be estimated by blood flow, whereas the majority of metastatic sites is determined by the specific local microenvironment for specific metastasis (Paget's "seed and soil" hypothesis, 1889) [43–45]. Tumor cells metastasize into the best vascularized parts of the skeleton, particularly the red bone marrow of the axial skeleton and the proximal ends of the long bones, the rips, and the vertebral column. Hematologic malignancies (e.g., myeloma, Hodgkin's disease) and solid tumors (e.g., breast, prostate) share the same bone-spreading pattern. Skeletal metastasis can cause substantial morbidity, including pain, pathologic fractures, neurological deficits, anemia and hypercalcemia secondary to osteoclastic activity and immobilization. Skeletal metastases are classified into predominantly osteoblastic, osteolytic, or mixed-type metastasis.

At present, treatment of bone pain from metastasis remains palliative [46–48]. Standard therapy includes systemic analgesics, antitumoral agents, hormones, bisphosphonates, chemotherapy, steroids, local surgery, anesthesia, and external beam radiation [49].

In osteoblastic and mixed-type metastasis, systemic radioisotope therapy with strontium-89, samarium-153, rhenium-186, or rhenium-188 seems to be an alternative [49–51]. All radioisotopes are β-emitters with a penetration of a few millimeters, which accumulate in the surrounding hyperactive bone tissue and not in the cancer cells. Due to accumulation in hyperactive bone, this technique is limited to osteoblastic and mixed-type metastasis (e.g., prostate and breast cancer).

10.3.1 Thermoablation

Thermoablation should be reserved for patients with osteolytic or mixed-type painful bone metastasis who are not suitable candidates for or have failed other standard forms of therapy. Furthermore, patients who have recurrent pain at a previous irradiated site and may not be eligible for secondary radiotherapy or surgery. Patients with recurrent pain after thermoablation could be treated a second time by thermoablation if an acceptable pain-free or pain-reduced interval can been achieved. The patient's pain must be from a solitary site of metastatic bone disease.

Current cross-sectional imaging (magnetic resonance imaging [MRI] or computed tomography [CT]) is essential for therapy planning.

The severity of pain (visual analogue pain scale [VAS], Brief Pain Inventory [BPI], Memorial Pain Assessment Card), life quality (International Quality-of-Life Assessment [IQOLA], Quality-of-Life Questionnaire [QLQ-C30]), and analgesics, especially morphine use (morphine equivalent dose) should be carefully determined before therapy to investigate outcome after therapy [52–55] (Fig. 10.2).

Analog to thermal ablation of osteoid osteoma spinal lesions or lesions near neural elements should be excluded from thermotherapy or, in experienced hands, treated with extreme care. Additionally, metastasis with contact to hollow viscera should not be treated with thermoablation.

Lesions in weight-bearing bones can be treated only if there is a low risk for a pathologic fracture. Mirels's scoring system for metastatic bone disease is an easy-to-use system for estimating the risk of a pathologic fracture (Table 10.2)

Table 10.2 Mirels's scoring system for metastatic bone disease. If lesion scores ≥ 8, prophylactic fixation is recommended [56]

Variable	1	2	3
Site	Upper limb	Lower limb	Peritrochanteric
Pain	Mild	Moderate	Functional
Lesion	Blastic	Mixed	Lytic
Size[a]	< 1/3	1/3–2/3	> 2/3

[a] As seen on plain X-ray, maximum destruction of cortex in any view

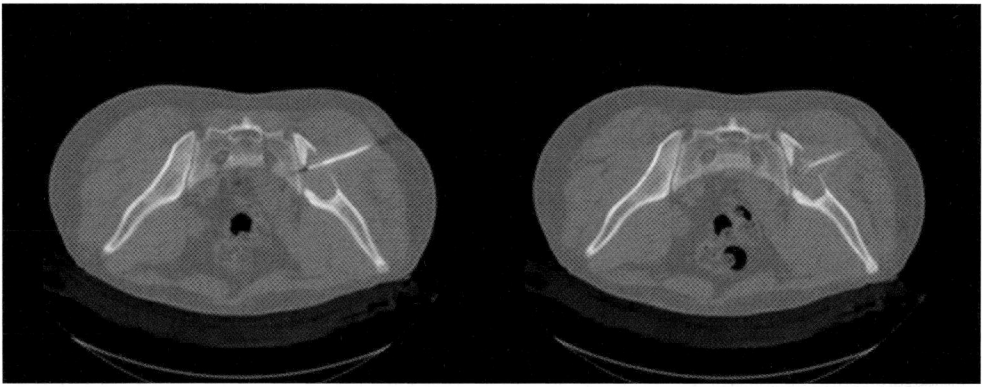

Fig. 10.2 Thermal ablation of an iliac skeletal metastasis by radiofrequency ablation (RFA)

[56]. In lesions scoring 8 or more, a prophylactic orthopedic fixation of the metastasis is recommended. For the intervention, a severe coagulation disorder should be excluded and a platelet count of 50 000/µl or higher and an international normalized ratio (INR) of 2 or greater were required prior to intervention (Fig. 10.3).

In hypervascular skeletal metastasis, often in renal cancer, a preinterventional transcatheter embolization with microparticles facilitates thermoablation, because high blood flow will cause convective cooling during the procedure and thus a longer time will be necessary for ablation or smaller and incomplete necrosis will result.

Potential complications of thermal ablation include hemorrhage, infection, nerve damage, fracture, and skin burning. Depending on the lesion location, transient bowel or bladder incontinence and paraplegia in spinal lesions could result. In radiofrequency ablation, additional skin burning at the site of the ground pads can occur.

Skeletal metastasis could be treated by thermoablation under conscious sedation or general anesthesia, depending on investigator's and/or patient's demand. For conscious sedation, we prefer analgosedation with midazolam and fentanyl under continuous ECG and oxygen-saturation monitoring. Additional local anesthetics (e.g., lidocaine) were administered at the skin entrance and at the periosteum prior to intervention.

LITT and RFA are the most frequently used techniques in thermal ablation of skeletal lesions. In water-cooled LITT, a 9F applicator tip needs to be placed in the center of the lesion, which could be facilitated by power-drilling, especially in osteoblastic skeletal lesions. Usually the laser beam is transmitted by a fiber with a 2-cm diffuser tip and 5 W of energy per active centimeter length for 6–8 min. In LITT, the temperature of the lesion and the surrounding tissues could be monitored with dedicated temperature-sensitive sequences in MRI.

In radiofrequency ablation, depending on the device used, the diameter of the applicator is usually smaller and placement especially in osteolytic metastasis is easier compared to LITT. If there is an indication for ablation in osteoblastic metastasis power-drilling is mandatory in RFA and LITT. The target temperature is usually 100°C, which should be maintained for 5–15 min. In smaller lesions (≤3 cm), a single ablation is typically adequate. Larger lesions require a second ablation to ensure tumor cell destruction, best combined with an applicator replacement. The emphasis on thermal treatment in larger lesions should be the tumor–bone interface, because pain often originates from this area due to nerval infiltration and osteoclastic activity.

Dupuy et al. first reported thermal ablation for symptomatic skeletal metastasis in ten patients with persistent pain despite prior external-beam radiation or chemotherapy [57]. In nine of ten patients, the Memorial Pain Assessment Card showed attenuation of pain. Besides case reports, five larger series with thermoablation in skeletal metastasis have been published. All showed pain relief in previously treated patients and therefore thermal ablation seems to be a practical alternative for this group of patients.

After skeletal bone thermoablation, immedi-

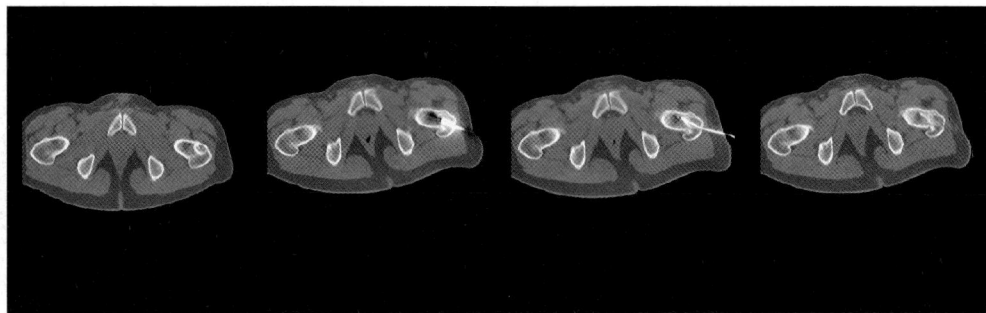

Fig. 10.3 Thermal ablation of a femoral metastasis from a follicular thyroid carcinoma by LITT. CT-guided power drilling and guidewire placement. Introduction of the laser fiber and thermal destruction

Table 10.3 Studies published concerning thermoablation in symptomatic skeletal metastasis with failed response to standard therapy

Author	Patients	Therapy	Previous therapy	Lesion diameter	Assessment	Change
Dupuy 1998 et al. [57]	10	RFA	Rx, Ch	1–8 cm	MPAC	Attenuation in 9/10 patients
Callstrom et al. 2002 [85]	12	RFA	Rx, Ch	1–11 cm	BPI	BPI: 8,0 → 2.4 (4 weeks)
Goetz et al. 2004 [86]	43	RFA	Rx, Ag	1–18 cm	BPI	BPI: 7,9 → 1.4 (12 weeks)
Friedl et al. 2004 [60]	10	RFA	Rx, Ch, Ag	NS	VAS, IQOLA-S36, QLQ-C30	VAS: 6,0 → 1.0 (6 weeks)
Grönemeyer et al. 2002 [87]	10	RFA + vertebroplasty (n = 4)	Rx, Ch, Ag	1.5–9 cm	VAS, HFAQ, Frankel score	VAS: 6,0 → 2.6 (mean, 5.8 months)

Rx, radiation therapy; Ch, chemotherapy; Ag, analgesic therapy; BPI, Brief Pain Inventory; MPAC, Memorial Pain Assessment Card; VAS, Visual Analog Scale; HFAQ, Hannover Functional Ability Questionnaire

ate pain reduction is typical, whereas in standard radiation therapy the maximal analgesic effect requires up to 20 weeks [58, 59].

Physiological mechanisms of pain reduction resulting from thermal ablation in skeletal metastasis are inhibition of signal transduction due to physical destruction of sensory nerves in the periosteum or corticalis, reduction of tumor volume with decompression and reduced stimulus for pain fibers, changes in the local microenvironment (e.g., reduction of osteoclastic and nerve-stimulating cytokines such as interleukins and TNF-alpha), and destruction of osteoclasts [60].

Thermoablation can be combined with other microtherapies, even in the same session. Combination with percutaneous cement injection (analog to cementoplasty or vertebroplasty) is common [61–64]. In this technique, liquid bone cement, e.g., polymethyl-methacrylate, is injected through a dedicated cannula into the trabecular structure of the bone. Painful microfractures of the osteolytic bone should be prevented due to stabilization of the bone; whether pathologic fractures can be prevented with this technique remains unclear. Furthermore, it is postulated that exothermal hardening of the bone cement has a cytotoxic effect on regional tumor cells.

Another therapeutic approach is the combination of thermal ablation and local cytotoxic drug injection. As cytotoxic drugs, high-concentrated ethanol, chemotherapeuticals such as Novantrone or liposomal doxorubicin, and cytokine antagonists (TNF-alpha-antagonists) have been investigated or still are under investigation [65–69].

Another therapeutic approach is CT-guided brachytherapy of symptomatic skeletal metastasis, but no larger series concerning this technique have been published so far [70].

In conclusion, thermal ablative therapy is an advancing alternative in osteoid osteomas. Thermal therapy is a minimally invasive therapy that reduces invasiveness compared to conventional surgery and shortens hospital stays and rehabilitation for the patient.

In case of failure of standard therapy in symptomatic bone metastasis, thermal ablation seems to be an alternative in palliative intention (Table 10.3).

The safety and results of this technique in the spine, especially in the posterior aspect of the vertebral body, are unclear. Treatment in this area should be restricted to experienced users.

References

1. Rhim H, Goldberg SN, Dodd GD 3rd et al. (2001) Essential techniques for successful radio-frequency thermal ablation of malignant hepatic tumors. Radiographics 21:S17–S35; discussion S36–S39
2. Goldberg SN, Gazelle GS, Mueller PR (2000) Thermal ablation therapy for focal malignancy: a unified approach to underlying principles, techniques, and diagnostic imaging guidance. AJR Am J Roentgenol 174:323–331
3. Ahmed M, Liu Z, Afzal KS et al. (2004) Radiofrequency ablation: effect of surrounding tissue composition on coagulation necrosis in a canine tumor model. Radiology 230:761–767
4. Vogl TJ, Mack MG, Muller PK et al. (1999) Interventional MR: interstitial therapy. Eur Radiol 9:1479–1487
5. Matsumoto R, Selig AM, Colucci VM et al. (1992) Interstitial Nd:YAG laser ablation in normal rabbit liver: trial to maximize the size of laser-induced lesions. Lasers Surg Med 12:650–658
6. Vogl TJ, Mack MG, Roggan A et al. (1998) Internally cooled power laser for MR-guided interstitial laser-induced thermotherapy of liver lesions: initial clinical results. Radiology 209:381–385
7. Organ LW (1976) Electrophysiologic principles of radiofrequency lesion making. Appl Neurophysiol 39:69–76
8. Goldberg SN, Dupuy DE (2001) Image-guided radiofrequency tumor ablation: challenges and opportunities – part I. J Vasc Interv Radiol 12:1021–1032
9. Dupuy DE, Goldberg SN (2001) Image-guided radiofrequency tumor ablation: challenges and opportunities – part II. J Vasc Interv Radiol 12:1135–1148
10. Goldberg SN, Gazelle GS, Dawson SL et al. (1995) Tissue ablation with radiofrequency using multiprobe arrays. Acad Radiol 2:670–674
11. Livraghi T, Goldberg SN, Monti F et al. (1997) Saline-enhanced radio-frequency tissue ablation in the treatment of liver metastases. Radiology 202:205–210
12. Miao Y, Ni Y, Yu J et al. (2001) An ex vivo study on radiofrequency tissue ablation: increased lesion size by using an "expandable-wet" electrode. Eur Radiol 11:1841–1847
13. Lencioni R, Goletti O, Armillotta N et al. (1998) Radio-frequency thermal ablation of liver metastases with a cooled-tip electrode needle: results of a pilot clinical trial. Eur Radiol 8:1205–1211
14. Anderson RL, Kapp DS (1990) Hyperthermia in cancer therapy: current status. Med J Aust 152:310–315
15. Nath S, Haines DE (1995) Biophysics and pathology of catheter energy delivery systems. Prog Cardiovasc Dis 37:185–204
16. Kennedy JE, Ter Haar GR, Cranston D (2003) High intensity focused ultrasound: surgery of the future? Br J Radiol 76:590–599
17. Kennedy JE (2005) High-intensity focused ultrasound in the treatment of solid tumours. Nat Rev Cancer 5:321–327
18. Wu F, Wang ZB, Chen WZ et al. (2004) Extracorporeal focused ultrasound surgery for treatment of human solid carcinomas: early Chinese clinical experience. Ultrasound Med Biol 30:245–260
19. Jaffe HL (1935) Osteoid osteoma: a benign osteoblastic tumor composed of osteoid and atypical bone. Arch Surg 31:709–728
20. Mungo DV, Zhang X, O'Keefe RJ et al. (2002) COX-1 and COX-2 expression in osteoid osteomas. J Orthop Res 20:159–162
21. Sim FH, Dahlin CD, Beabout JW (1975) Osteoid-osteoma: diagnostic problems. J Bone Joint Surg Am 57:154–159
22. Campanacci M, Ruggieri P, Gasbarrini A et al. (1999) Osteoid osteoma. Direct visual identification and intralesional excision of the nidus with minimal removal of bone. J Bone Joint Surg Br 81:814–820
23. Kneisl JS, Simon MA (1992) Medical management compared with operative treatment for osteoid osteoma. J Bone Joint Surg Am 74:179–185
24. Marcove RC, Heelan RT, Huvos AG et al. (1991) Osteoid osteoma. Diagnosis, localization, and treatment. Clin Orthop Relat Res 267:197–201
25. Rosenthal DI, Hornicek FJ, Wolfe MW et al. (1998) Percutaneous radiofrequency coagulation of osteoid osteoma compared with operative treatment. J Bone Joint Surg Am 80:815–821
26. Pfeiffer M, Sluga M, Windhager R et al. (2003) Surgical treatment of osteoid osteoma of the extremities. Z Orthop Ihre Grenzgeb 141:345–348
27. Sluga M, Windhager R, Pfeiffer M et al. (2002) Peripheral osteoid osteoma. Is there still a place for traditional surgery? J Bone Joint Surg Br 84:249–251

28. Rosenthal DI, Alexander A, Rosenberg AE et al. (1992) Ablation of osteoid osteomas with a percutaneously placed electrode: a new procedure. Radiology 183:29–33
29. Binkert CA, Nanz D, Bootz F et al. (2002) Laser-induced thermotherapy of the vertebral body: preliminary assessment of safety and real-time magnetic resonance monitoring in an animal model. Invest Radiol 37:557–561
30. Cove JA, Taminiau AH, Obermann WR et al. (2000) Osteoid osteoma of the spine treated with percutaneous computed tomography-guided thermocoagulation. Spine 25:1283–1286
31. Gangi A, Basille A, Buy X et al. (2005) Radiofrequency and laser ablation of spinal lesions. Semin Ultrasound CT MR 26:89–97
32. Samaha EI, Ghanem IB, Moussa RF et al. (2005) Percutaneous radiofrequency coagulation of osteoid osteoma of the "Neural Spinal Ring". Eur Spine J 14:702–705
33. Hadjipavlou AG, Lander PH, Marchesi D et al. (2003) Minimally invasive surgery for ablation of osteoid osteoma of the spine. Spine 28: E472–E477
34. Erdtmann B, Duda SH, Pereira P et al. (2001) CT-guided therapy of osteoid osteoma by drill trepanation of the nidus. Clinical follow-up results. Rofo Fortschr Geb Rontgenstr Neuen Bildgeb Verfahr 173:708–713
35. Klose KC, Forst R, Vorwerk D et al. (1991) The percutaneous removal of osteoid osteomas via CT-guided drilling. Rofo Fortschr Geb Rontgenstr Neuen Bildgeb Verfahr 155:532–537
36. Kohler R, Rubini J, Postec F et al. (1995) Treatment of osteoid osteoma by CT-controlled percutaneous drill resection. Apropos of 27 cases. Rev Chir Orthop Reparatrice Appar Mot 81:317–325
37. Adam G, Neuerburg J, Vorwerk D et al. (1997) Percutaneous treatment of osteoid osteomas: combonation of drill biopsy and subsequent ethanol injection. Semin Musculoskelet Radiol 1:281–284
38. Sanhaji L, Gharbaoui IS, Hassani RE et al. (1996) A new treatment of osteoid osteoma: percutaneous sclerosis with ethanol under scanner guidance. J Radiol 77:37–40
39. Duda SH, Schnatterbeck P, Harer T et al. (1997) Treatment of osteoid osteoma with CT-guided drilling and ethanol instillation. Dtsch Med Wochenschr 122:507–510
40. Baker RC, Kramer RE (1999) Cytotoxicity of short-chain alcohols. Annu Rev Pharmacol Toxicol 39:127–150
41. Jemal A, Thomas A, Murray T et al. (2002) Cancer statistics, 2002. CA Cancer J Clin 52:23–47
42. Jemal A, Murray T, Ward E et al. (2005) Cancer statistics, 2005. CA Cancer J Clin 55:10–30
43. Paget S (1889) The distribution of secondary growths in cancer of the breast. Lancet 1:571–573
44. Liotta LA, Kohn E (1990) Cancer invasion and metastases. JAMA 263:1123–1126
45. Woodhouse EC, Chuaqui RF, Liotta LA (1997) General mechanisms of metastasis. Cancer 80 [8 Suppl]:1529–1537
46. Nielsen OS (1996) Palliative treatment of bone metastases. Acta Oncol 35 [Suppl 5]:58–60
47. Nielsen OS, Munro AJ, Tannock IF (1991) Bone metastases: pathophysiology and management policy. J Clin Oncol 9:509–524
48. Campa JA 3rd, Payne R (1992) The management of intractable bone pain: a clinician's perspective. Semin Nucl Med 22:3–10
49. Serafini AN (2001) Therapy of metastatic bone pain. J Nucl Med 42:895–906
50. Serafini AN, Houston SJ, Resche I et al. (1998) Palliation of pain associated with metastatic bone cancer using samarium-153 lexidronam: a double-blind placebo-controlled clinical trial. J Clin Oncol 16:1574–1581
51. Palmedo H, Manka-Waluch A, Albers P et al. (2003) Repeated bone-targeted therapy for hormone-refractory prostate carcinoma: tandomized phase II trial with the new, high-energy radiopharmaceutical rhenium-188 hydroxyethylidenediphosphonate. J Clin Oncol 21:2869–2875
52. Aaronson NK, Ahmedzai S, Bergman B et al. (1993) The European Organization for Research and Treatment of Cancer QLQ-C30: a quality-of-life instrument for use in international clinical trials in oncology. J Natl Cancer Inst 85:365–376
53. Pereira J, Lawlor P, Vigano A et al. (2001) Equianalgesic dose ratios for opioids. A critical review and proposals for long-term dosing. J Pain Symptom Manage 22:672–687
54. Ware JE Jr, Gandek B (1998) Overview of the SF-36 Health Survey and the International Quality of Life Assessment (IQOLA) Project. J Clin Epidemiol 51:903–912

55. Daut RL, Cleeland CS, Flanery RC (1983) Development of the Wisconsin Brief Pain Questionnaire to assess pain in cancer and other diseases. Pain 17:197–210
56. Mirels H (1989) Metastatic disease in long bones. A proposed scoring system for diagnosing impending pathologic fractures. Clin Orthop Relat Res 249:256–264
57. Dupuy DE, Safran H, Mayo-Smith WW et al. (1998) Radiofrequency ablation of painful osseous metastases (abstract). Radiology 202 [Suppl]:389
58. Janjan N (2001) Bone metastases: approaches to management. Semin Oncol 28 [4 Suppl 11]:28–34
59. Janjan NA (1997) Radiation for bone metastases: conventional techniques and the role of systemic radiopharmaceuticals. Cancer 80 [8 Suppl]:1628–1645
60. Friedl G, Tauss J, Portugaller RH et al. (2004) Die perkutane Radiofrequenzablation (PRFA) bei symptomatischen sekundär-neoplastischen Knochenläsionen. Z Orthop Ihre Grenzgeb 142:727–734
61. Schaefer O, Lohrmann C, Herling M et al. (2002) Combined radiofrequency thermal ablation and percutaneous cementoplasty treatment of a pathologic fracture. J Vasc Interv Radiol 13:1047–1050
62. Schaefer O, Lohrmann C, Markmiller M et al. (2003) Technical innovation. Combined treatment of a spinal metastasis with radiofrequency heat ablation and vertebroplasty. AJR Am J Roentgenol 180:1075–1077
63. Cotten A, Demondion X, Boutry N et al. (1999) Therapeutic percutaneous injections in the treatment of malignant acetabular osteolyses. Radiographics 19:647–653
64. Cotten A, Boutry N, Cortet B et al. (1998) Percutaneous vertebroplasty: state of the art. Radiographics 18:311–320; discussion 320–313
65. Gangi A, Dietemann JL, Schultz A et al. (1996) Interventional radiologic procedures with CT guidance in cancer pain management. Radiographics 16:1289–1304; discussion 1304–1306
66. Ahmed M, Liu Z, Lukyanov AN et al. (2005) Combination radiofrequency ablation with intratumoral liposomal doxorubicin: effect on drug accumulation and coagulation in multiple tissues and tumor types in animals. Radiology 235:469–477
67. Goldberg SN, Saldinger PF, Gazelle GS et al. (2001) Percutaneous tumor ablation: increased necrosis with combined radio-frequency ablation and intratumoral doxorubicin injection in a rat breast tumor model. Radiology 220:420–427
68. Gronemeyer DH, Seibel RM (1993) Mikroinvasive CT-gesteuerte Tumortherapie von Weichteil- und Sklettmetastasen. Wien Med Wochenschr 143:312–321
69. Tobinick EL (2003) Targeted etanercept for treatment-refractory pain due to bone metastasis: two case reports. Clin Ther 25:2279–2288
70. Kolotas C, Baltas D, Zamboglou N (1999) CT-based interstitial HDR brachytherapy. Strahlenther Onkol 175:419–427
71. Rosenthal DI, Hornicek FJ, Torriani M et al. (2003) Osteoid osteoma: percutaneous treatment with radiofrequency energy. Radiology 229:171–175
72. Rimondi E, Bianchi G, Malaguti MC et al. (2005) Radiofrequency thermoablation of primary non-spinal osteoid osteoma: optimization of the procedure. Eur Radiol 15:1393–1399
73. Vanderschueren GM, Taminiau AH, Obermann WR et al. (2002) Osteoid osteoma: clinical results with thermocoagulation. Radiology 224:82–86
74. Lindner NJ, Ozaki T, Roedl R et al. (2001) Percutaneous radiofrequency ablation in osteoid osteoma. J Bone Joint Surg Br 83:391–396
75. Woertler K, Vestring T, Boettner F et al. (2001) Osteoid osteoma: CT-guided percutaneous radiofrequency ablation and follow-up in 47 patients. J Vasc Interv Radiol 12:717–722
76. Cioni R, Armillotta N, Bargellini I et al. (2004) CT-guided radiofrequency ablation of osteoid osteoma: long-term results. Eur Radiol 14:1203–1208
77. Gangi A, Dietemann JL, Clavert JM et al. (1998) Treatment of osteoid osteoma using laser photocoagulation. Apropos of 28 cases. Rev Chir Orthop Reparatrice Appar Mot 84:676–684
78. Witt JD, Hall-Craggs MA, Ripley P et al. (2000) Interstitial laser photocoagulation for the treatment of osteoid osteoma. J Bone Joint Surg Br 82:1125–1128
79. Ghanem I, Collet LM, Kharrat K et al. (2003) Percutaneous radiofrequency coagulation of osteoid osteoma in children and adolescents. J Pediatr Orthop B 12:244–252

80. Gebauer B, Tunn PU, Gaffke G et al. (2005) Osteoid osteoma: experience with laser- and radiofrequency-induced ablation. Cardiovasc Intervent Radiol 29:210–215
81. Gallazzi MB, Arborio G, Garbagna PG et al. (2001) Percutaneous radio-frequency ablation of osteoid osteoma: technique and preliminary results. Radiol Med (Torino) 102:329–334
82. Barei DP, Moreau G, Scarborough MT et al. (2000) Percutaneous radiofrequency ablation of osteoid osteoma. Clin Orthop Relat Res 373:115–124
83. Venbrux AC, Montague BJ, Murphy KP et al. (2003) Image-guided percutaneous radiofrequency ablation for osteoid osteomas. J Vasc Interv Radiol 14:375–380
84. Sequeiros RB, Hyvonen P, Sequeiros AB et al. (2003) MR imaging-guided laser ablation of osteoid osteomas with use of optical instrument guidance at 0.23 T. Eur Radiol 13:2309–2314
85. Callstrom MR, Charboneau JW, Goetz MP et al. (2002) Painful metastases involving bone: feasibility of percutaneous CT- and US-guided radiofrequency ablation. Radiology 224:87–97
86. Goetz MP, Callstrom MR, Charboneau JW et al. (2004) Percutaneous image-guided radiofrequency ablation of painful metastases involving bone: a multicenter study. J Clin Oncol 22:300–306
87. Gronemeyer DH, Schirp S, Gevargez A (2002) Image-guided radiofrequency ablation of spinal tumors: preliminary experience with an expandable array electrode. Cancer J 8:33–39